# CONTROLLING HORMONES NATURALLY

*My Journey For Solutions To PMS, Menopause & Osteoporosis with Wild Yam*

*By*

## MELINDA BONK

MB Publishers, Minneapolis

Contact:
Melinda Bonk
MB Publishers
2101 Kennedy Street, NE, Suite 307
Minneapolis, MN 55413
(612) 378-8830

ISBN 0-96508-270-9
First Edition 1996
Printed in the United States of America

Medical Editor: Lauri M. Aesoph, N.D.
Copy Editor: Laura Kath Fraser
Cover Graphics & Book Design: Patrick Redmond
Typesetting: Mori Studio

# Dedication

This Book Is Dedicated To My Family

*A journey of a thousand miles*
*must begin with a single step.*
*~Lao-Tzu*

# Acknowledgements

MY SINCERE THANKS GO to the many people who have inspired me to write this book. I especially want to thank all the health care practitioners who helped find solutions to my health problems as well as educated me along the journey.

To my medical editor, Dr. Lauri Aesoph, for making sure all the important medical background information was presented correctly, and could be easily understand by women and men of all ages.

To my copy editor, Laura Kath Fraser, whose enthusiasm and support kept me going and made this readable.

Finally, I would like to extend my heartfelt appreciation to all the wonderful women who shared their personal journeys and success stories about controlling their hormones with the wild yam.

# Table of Contents

# *Introduction*

# A Very Personal Note About My Journey Of Discovery

I LEARNED HOW TO control hormones naturally when I discovered the wild yam and healed my PMS. As I traveled the rocky road of recovery, I learned valuable information that gave me back my health and happiness.

Generations of women have neglected to talk about their bodies. My mother never prepared me mentally or emotionally for the dramatic hormonal shifts we shared as women—beginning with menstruation in puberty, the opportunity of pregnancy during our teens through our forties, and lastly, menopause. I didn't have a clue how important hormones are to women, or the relationship they play in our lives.

## Is This All In My Mind?

Like so many women, I have suffered from an arsenal of physical and emotional symptoms around my menstrual cycle. Years of anger, tears, depression, irritability and mood swings—pre-menstrual syndrome (PMS)—raised havoc in my life. The breast tenderness, fatigue and cramps seemed endless, as if I had a flu that wouldn't go away.

As I entered my thirties and experienced stressful changes in jobs, husbands, boyfriends and cities, my PMS symptoms became more pronounced. I went to the local drug store for quick rescue remedies like Midol™ or Motrin™, but they didn't cure my problems. In my ignorance, I unwisely considered these symptoms to be a natural part of womanhood, or perhaps just in my head. With menopause right around the corner, what could I expect then?

Finally, my never-ending, extreme ailments led me to see my family doctor. I was sick and tired of being sick and tired. So, you can imagine my surprise, when, after a complete physical exam and blood tests, my doctor told me I was normal. I didn't understand how I could feel that bad and still be handed a clean bill of health. For lack of answers to my complaints, the only prescription my doctor offered was...rest.

## Traveling In A New World

When all else fails, go for rest and relaxation! What could be better for my health than a warm sunny beach in Florida and some of Mom's chicken soup? While visiting her, I met Burton Goldberg, a book publisher who specializes in alternative medicine. Fortunately, he opened my eyes to a new world of natural medicine and healing. At a time when I was so sick, it was fateful that he introduced me to doctors practicing natural medicine. I had no idea they even existed! Until then, I had been the typical patient and consumer. If I was slightly sick, I went to a drug store. If I felt deathly ill, I'd see a doctor for a prescription. This was the only medicine I knew, until the world of natural medicine opened up to me. Conventional medicine had let me down, and I desperately needed new answers. Since I was not yet ready to trust my health to doctors of any kind, I was filled with skeptical questions. What was natural medicine? Who were these doctors? Could they help me?

Courageously, I began a journey that answered my questions and transformed my life. I discovered types of doctors that blended natural ancient remedies with modern medical techniques. For example, these physicians used the latest diagnostic methods such as blood tests and CAT scans, yet turned to Mother Nature for most of their treatments—like the use of herbs and homeopathy. I found out that natural medicine isn't hocus pocus or quackery, but rather sensible, time-tested therapies to help your body heal. While conventional medicine shut me out with no answers, natural medicine opened the door that ended my suffering.

## New Discoveries

It could hardly be a coincidence that the first doctor I met on my journey to discover natural solutions was an expert on women's health. John R. Lee, M.D., of Sebastopol, California, author of *Natural Progesterone: The Multiple Roles of A Remarkable Hormone,* has had successful results treating women's hormone problems with natural progesterone made from the wild yam since 1982. I was intrigued and inspired when I learned that Dr. Lee has helped women overcome PMS, menstrual problems and menopausal symptoms (like hot flashes and night sweats), as well as preventing osteoporosis.

After reading his numerous research papers on natural progesterone, I learned that a woman's health depends on how well her hormones are balanced by each other. Throughout the special stages of womanhood—puberty, pregnancy and menopause—estrogen and progesterone are constantly fluctuating up and down monthly. It's when this balancing act fumbles and one hormone overshoots normal levels that problems can begin.

One day, a light went off in my head. My troubles weren't in my head, they were in my hormones! At that moment, the wise woman within began to open my eyes and my mind to natural options. Natural progesterone from the wild yam could be my salvation. While editing my first book on natural medicine, I spoke with many natural health practitioners. They all echoed what Dr. Lee had told me. Natural progesterone from the wild yam not only could help my PMS, could relieve menopausal symptoms and a number of other hormone-based female conditions. Natural progesterone could even replace Estrogen Replacement Therapy (ERT) and other synthetic hormone treatments.

Why didn't my regular medical doctor (M.D.) tell me about these natural solutions? The more I questioned practitioners, the more I noticed differences between types of doctors and their treatments. I realized that M.D.'s don't know it all and they really can't fix everything. These natural health discoveries were startling news to me (and unknown to my family medical doctor), but these solutions are old news to the people who practice them. Natural medicine is not a fad—its treatments are centuries old—and, I might add, here to stay. I also discovered many conventional health professionals who have embraced natural medical knowledge and incorporated these safe and effective therapies into their practices. The reality of my discovery is yesterday's medicine is today's alternative.

## Wellness Restored

Gradually, I switched from pills to plants with the information I discovered along my journey. Before I tried any natural therapies, I took what I had learned and developed some theories of my own. Since natural progesterone, which is derived from the wild yam, helps so many health problems, I wondered if wild yam alone could achieve the same results. I launched a wellness plan using wild yam cream, diet changes and vitamin and mineral supplements. The road to health was a long process. It didn't occur in a week or two, as I was accustomed to with conventional medicine. Healing takes time. After all, it took a long while for my health to decline. Eventually, I regained my health and felt great once again. The wild yam and other treatments I used were safer, cheaper and more effective than the estrogen, anti-depressants and diuretics I'd tried. My new health plan cured my PMS problems, not just masked the symptoms. The wild yam has made a dramatic, positive difference in my life. I finally feel at peace and happy.

After I cured my PMS, I badgered my sister, who had menopausal problems, to get off her ERT and try wild yam cream. She did and the results were amazing. Within five months, her symptoms were gone and she was her old self again. It seemed wild yam cream could help smooth out the menopause transition and solve other hormone problems. Natural progesterone derived from the wild yam could help osteoporosis (simplistically, the loss of bone density as we age), too!

# Why This Book?

I am passionate about conveying this message to every woman—there ARE natural solutions for relieving PMS, menopause and preventing osteoporosis! Synthetic hormone pills and drug therapies are not the only way! My mission is to let you know that you do not have to suffer any more hormone imbalances, or be at risk of developing osteoporosis. You can learn, as I did, which natural solutions are available.

As an average consumer, I really felt that I needed to understand everything I could about natural medicine, herbs, hormones and the risks and benefits of Hormone Replacement Therapy (HRT). Then, I could make an intelligent decision about my health and my life. I want to save you the time, energy and frustration that I experienced on the path to controlling your hormones and controlling your life.

I wrote this book with the hope that by sharing my discoveries, you can make intelligent choices for yourself. Each one of us is unique, in our body and our journey toward health. I hope each one of you opens your heart and listens to your own wise woman within.

# Just A Thought . . .

*Depression is not a Prozac™ deficiency.*
*Headaches are not an aspirin scarcity.*
*Since menopause cannot be solved with a Premarin™ tablet,*
*And osteoporosis won't straighten up with Os-Cal™...*
*Why do we run to pills for answers when*
*our bodies and Mother Nature have the solutions?*

*Part One*

# THE ROAD TO NATURAL SOLUTIONS

# Chapter 1

# NATURAL MEDICINE

WHEN I FIRST DISCOVERED that there was more to "medicine" than popping a pill, I was overwhelmed by the vast subject of "natural medicine." I was intrigued that herbs could solve my medical problems. I found it hard to imagine that a particular root, berry or leaf could heal my hormone woes. So I hunted for more knowledge. I learned that Mother Nature provides nutrients from food and medicines from plants. My skepticism around natural medicine decreased the more I understood that herbs—one of natural medicine's mainstays—as well as homeopathic remedies, derived in part from plants, have been used for centuries with outstanding results.

I'm sharing this background information about the use of herbs and homeopathy in natural medicine with you because I think that knowledge is power. If you understand some of the history, theory and practical applications of two important parts of natural medicine—herbs and homeopathy—then you have the power to find natural solutions to your medical problems. The power of understanding and the willingness to question and seek the truth will ultimately make you healthier, too. I found that to be true!

## Herbal History

The science and art of medicinal herbs for healing has been practiced from ancient times—over 5,000 years ago—to modern times. Most cultures have centuries of historical evidence that plants work for healing countless conditions. Traditional Chinese medicine is a 3,500 year old system that focuses on herbal remedies and acupuncture. The Egyptians first recorded the effects of plant medicine around 2,300 B.C.. Herbal medicine, once the top ranking form of medicine, is still the main source of medical assistance in many parts of the world today. This is because medicinal herbs provide safe, cheap and effective treatments for so many ailments. There has been a renewed interest in natural and herbal medicine during the past decade in the United States. This is primarily due to the rising cost of conventional health care services as well as health insurance, and a concern by many Americans about the safety of drugs and surgery. Natural therapies are viable options. The recently formed Office of Alternative Medicine, part of the National Institutes of Health (NIH) in Rockville, Maryland, is dedicated to studying the benefits of alternative medicine, from herbs to acupuncture to homeopathy. Over the past 15 years, there has been a worldwide renaissance of herbal medicine incorporating traditional wisdom from India, China, South America, Africa, Europe and Native American cultures.

## 5,000 Herbs And Counting

Although there are 300,000 to 500,000 plants known to humankind, only 5,000 have been studied for their medicinal applications. More researchers are discovering that certain compounds, called phytochemicals, in several plants have beneficial biochemical effects on the human body. (For example, the wild yam contains diosgenin.) The blueprints for many modern pharmaceutical drugs are these phytochemicals— some are synthetic versions, some are not. In fact, 121 prescription drugs (called allopathic medicines) come from only 90 species of plants, and 74 percent of these were discovered by following up native folklore claims.[1]

Pharmaceutical investigators, in their search for new cures, have revealed how the rest of these naturally occurring compounds affect the body. Many natural health practitioners, such as herbalists and naturopathic physicians, use herbs to treat several of the same conditions that M.D.'s treat with drugs, but without adverse effects. In addition, when herbs are used correctly, they also support the body during the healing process.

# Defining Herbal Medicine

We use plants or parts of plants every day—to make medicine, build our homes, for clothing, decorations, to flavor food or use as aromatic oils for soaps and fragrances. Depending on the plant, medicinal herbs include the leaf, flower, stem, seed, root, fruit or bark. In some cases, like *Sambucus nigra* or elder, different parts are used for different illnesses. Elder is considered a veritable medicine chest because its leaves heal wounds, the flowers are great for colds and the flu, and the berries are useful for rheumatism. Aloe Vera, that gelatinous plant this sits on kitchen sills all over the country, possesses amazing, wound healing abilities. The next time you burn yourself while cooking, just snap off a piece of aloe and apply it to your burn.

While many people still view herbs with skepticism, drugs and herbs are closely related. Pharmacognosy, a branch of pharmacology, bridges herbal medicine and modern medications. In fact, the science of pharmacognosy, known to some as phytochemistry, studies the physical characteristics and botanical sources of crude drugs. *Phyto* just means plant; *pharmaco* translates as drugs—two words describing basically the same thing—the study of plants for therapeutic purposes—but emphasizing a different side of the same spectrum. Herbal medicine is used to treat many health conditions. While I want to show you the benefits of wild yam for PMS, menopausal discomfort and other female complaints, there are herbs equally effective for insomnia, indigestion, heart disease, pain relief and a myriad of other acute and chronic diseases.

# The Big Difference Between Herbal And Allopathic Medicines

While herbs and allopathic medicines have similar modes of action, they have their differences, too. Do you remember the commercial— "It's not nice to fool Mother Nature!"—Well, she's not appreciative of what's happened to her herbs, either! A lone phytochemical can have healing properties. When it's isolated from a plant, much of what is good about that herbal medicine is lost. There are other constituents within a plant that interact with the "healing" phytochemical. When a whole plant is broken up into bits and pieces, this synergistic or cooperative interplay is lost. It would be like identifying a fantastic basketball player on a team, pulling her from the game and expecting her to perform as well alone as with her team mates. While she may still score many baskets, the support and cooperation from her team mates is lost.

The same scenario goes for phytochemicals yanked from an herb. They just don't work the same alone. When this same phytochemical is then synthesized or manufactured (versus using the natural form) and concentrated (we're talking about allopathic drugs here), more of the original herbal action is changed. For instance, side effects become a problem.

Herbs can be mixed together for even more benefits. These compounds may alter the individual actions of herbs, while increasing therapeutic effectiveness and reducing the chance of toxic side-effects. When used in the correct manner, herbal medicine strengthens the whole body, rather than suppressing symptoms. Some herbs also support and detoxify your body by removing toxins.

Herbs can be used allopathically, that is in the same manner that doctors prescribe most drugs—to relieve symptoms, but not cure. So if you have a cold, you can take the herb ephedra and the phytochemical ephedrine (similar in action to over-the-counter decongestants sold in drugstores) to dry up your stuffy nose. On the other hand, when herbs are taken to strengthen your body and roust its inner resources, then true healing occurs.

# Herbal Advantages

Used correctly, herbs are safe and effective with a minimum of side effects. I'm throwing a lot of information at you about what, for many of you, may be new and terrifying territory. So let's stop for a moment and review the advantages of herbs:

1. Herbs work on many of the body's systems to heal and regulate the body naturally.

2. Herbs have fewer (if any) side effects than synthetic drugs. In rare cases, you may experience an allergic reaction to an herb like a skin rash. On the other hand, the incidence of allergic reactions to drugs is not rare, and is in some cases, life-threatening.

3. When you treat a condition herbally, you generally use the whole plant in some form. Drugs usually use an isolated compound meant to work symptomatically.

4. When used properly, herbs solve the underlying problem of a disease by strengthening your body, not simply relieving the symptoms.

5.  When treating a condition with herbs, it may take longer to see results, but the goal is to reverse your problem for long-term benefits.
6.  Most herbs are non-addictive.

7.  Your body wants to heal itself. Herbs can complement that process, rather than deter it.

8.  Herbs nourish you with nutrients like vitamins and minerals, another plus in fighting disease; some herbs strengthen your immune system, too.

# Herbal Preparations

Herbal medicines are available in many different forms such as teas or tablets. Choose your preparation depending on your affliction, age, type of herb needed, the part of the herb being used and what is available. For example, sometimes you'll want a milder remedy, in which case a tea would do nicely. Perhaps you need a cream or poultice to treat a nasty cut. Plants are versatile, and so should you be when deciding the best form to use.

# Teas, Tisanes, Infusions And Decoctions

Probably the easiest way to use herbs are teas—to steep or boil all or part of the dried (or fresh) plant in water—not unlike the tea you drink for breakfast. Many health food stores or herbalist shops carry jars of dried herbs that have been cut up or powdered. You can also incorporate dried herbs into poultices or other herbal treatments for home use.

Herbal teas are also known as tisanes and come in either loose or tea bag form. Because of convenience, most Americans prefer tea bags. However, tea bags are pretty well restricted to infusions. Making an infusion is no different than brewing a nice "cup o' tea", by steeping the tea bag or loose tea in hot water for three to five minutes. This method is best suited for the leaves and flowers of an herb, parts of the plant that readily release their medicinal compounds and oh-so distinct aroma (sometimes pleasant, sometimes not).

There are times when you want to take advantage of a plant's healing bark or roots, not an easy fit in a tea bag. As you can imagine, these woody plant parts are harder to crack open for removal of medicinal ingredients. Decoctions are helpful for these types of plants. Put a couple teaspoons of your selected herb in a rolling boil of water for fifteen to twenty minutes, and sip the resulting beverage. That is a decoction.

# Capsules And Tablets

Pills are easy and clean to take, so it's no wonder that the most popular type of herbal medicine in the United States is capsules and tablets. Herbal capsules are generally stronger than teas and, unlike tea and other water-based extracts, offer your body all active constituents—not just the water soluble ones.

Herb pills are made like this: powdered herbs are placed in gelatin capsules or formed into tablets. The whole herb is used and requires minimal processing, so generally these pills are lower in cost than tinctures (see below). One drawback is the potency of herbal capsules changes over time because of oxygen, light and moisture exposure. Another potential problem is absorption of capsules and tablets. Fillers and binders used to make these pills can inhibit your body's ability to use the herbs. If your digestive tract isn't functioning up to snuff, this problem is compounded. One alternative is to use freeze-dried herbs in capsules instead, which are approximately four times stronger than regular powdered herbs.

# Tinctures

There are more plant constituents that are soluble in alcohol than water. This is where alcohol-based tinctures come into use. Because tinctures, like any form of alcohol, also contain water, you actually get both water and alcohol-soluble components. What else do tinctures have to offer? Well, they're quickly assimilated compared to pills and are more concentrated so you don't have to take as much (and storage is easier). One more thing, like those brandied pears you might make for Christmas presents, alcohol in an herbal tincture acts as a preservative. This means a longer shelf life for your herbal medicine. There are times, however, when you don't want to use tinctures because of their alcohol content. Don't give tinctures to children, recovering alcoholics, nursing or pregnant women. One way to get around this is to substitute a vinegar or glycerine type of tincture, or you can boil the alcohol off a tincture and use the residual liquid.

# Essential Oils

Don't you love the smell of lavender and eucalyptus? I do. Lavender reminds me of my grandmother and those little sachets she used to carry in her purse. Eucalyptus, the same smelly stuff found in chest rubs like Vicks Vapor Rub™, is great for easing your breathing during a cold or bronchitis. It is plants like these that contain volatile oils that are made into essential oils—the pure aromatic essences of herbs. You may be most familiar with essential oils as an additive to massage oils. A few drops of a fragrant oil in a potpourri or candle gives your home a pleasing smell. Several essential oils, like tea tree oil, have medicinal properties suitable for wounds, burns and other skin afflictions. Because essential oils are highly concentrated, they should be used with caution when applied to the skin. It's typical to dilute the essential herbal oil in a neutral base like olive oil.

# Salves, Ointments And Creams

Another way to treat external conditions like a gash or aching joint with herbs is with a salve, ointment or cream. Sometimes medicinal herbs are added to a cream for topical (on top of the skin) application. Salves and ointments range from pasty in appearance and texture to quite greasy, depending on their ingredients. Usually an oil, either vegetable or animal, is added to act as a carrier for the volatile oils you're trying to extract from the plant. They can also have a moisturizing effect. Wax is included to provide firmness. Gels are a new form of topical herbal medicines that absorb quickly.

# You Can't Patent A Plant

How do you patent garlic or ginger or wild yam? Pure food products and nutrients like vitamins or plants can't be patented because they're made by Mother Nature, not humans. Drugs can be patented and sold after the expensive clinical studies required by the Food & Drug Administration (FDA) are completed. The cost in developing a single new chemical compound for a drug can cost over $10 million over a 12 year period. Pharmaceutical companies agree to this process, because once finished, they own the marketing rights to whatever drugs they develop and test—a lucrative venture that more than pays back the high start-up costs.

Even though many pharmaceuticals originally came from plants, herbs don't make as much money. (Did you know many birth control pills are derived from the wild yam?) There is no profit incentive for businesses to spend millions of dollars to research the medicinal benefits of plant-based products, because their discoveries (and herbal products) can't be monopolized.

It's not just the scientists, it's doctors, too. The more I delved into research on natural medicine and hormones, the more I realized that most doctors don't have enough information about natural solutions to help women make informed choices. Many traditional doctors are closed to new information because they rely too heavily on standard medical journals and pharmaceutical companies for their medical updates (and most drug houses don't work with herbs). Although I am finding a lot more research on nutrition, herbs and other natural therapies in mainstream medical literature.

# Oh, And One More Thing...

Now that I've whetted your appetite for herbal medicine, I'm going to douse it a bit. Herbs are wonderful medicines and have saved my life. However, like buying any new product    for the first time, you need to educate yourself about the preparations you're buying. Not all formulas are created equal. This next lesson will merely add more information along your journey.

The efficacy and potency of an herb is also dependent on the quality, the skill used in preparing it, the storage method, the time of year it was harvested and the location of the harvest. When selecting an herb for a specific problem, be aware of what species you need. Some herbs, such as wild yam for instance, have several different species with differing medicinal value. Unlike some European countries, the United States doesn't regulate herbal quality or even precision. Korean ginseng or Panax ginseng, is a case in point. Studies have revealed that the active ingredient, ginsenoside, varies widely among commercial ginseng products. Some supposed ginseng preparations don't even contain ginseng![2]

# A Primer On Homeopathy

My main purpose in writing this book is to tell you about the wonderful healing qualities of the wild yam and my experiences using this natural herb. However, during my wellness journey, I discovered another powerful system of natural medicine called homeopathy. While just starting to gain substantial recognition in the United States, this low-cost, easy-to-use, non-toxic system of medicine is used by millions of people around the world.

Homeopathy is practiced by many kinds of trained professionals—medical doctors, herbalists, chiropractors, naturopathic physicians, osteopathic doctors and acupuncturists. With a little knowledge, you, too, can use homeopathy for mild ailments like a cold, or as an adjunct to your first aid kit. Practitioners report that homeopathy is very effective in treating chronic conditions as well as the more acute symptoms of everyday conditions like the flu. Because of its wide ranging effects, homeopathy is a logical first choice for almost any ailment before taking a synthetic drug. Consult with a trained homeopathic practitioner to do this.

## A Tried And True Therapy

The philosophy of homeopathy is far from new. In fact, Hippocrates and Parcelsus knew of its principles long ago. It wasn't until 1810 that modern homeopathy was born, when a German physician, Samuel Hahnemann, M.D., published *The Organon of Medicine*. This classic work established the experimental and theoretical basis of homeopathy in a systematic and scientific fashion.

Dr. Hahnemann's discovery came through his investigation of cinchona, a known herbal cure for malaria. He learned that when he took a large dose of cinchona, he suffered from the same symptoms as a malaria patient. His symptoms disappeared when he stopped taking cinchona. Dr. Hahnemann theorized that if taking a large dose of cinchona created malarial symptoms in a healthy person, then a minute amount of the same herb might cure a person suffering from malaria by stimulating the body's natural urge to fight disease. In other words, the same substance that produces the symptoms of an illness, can, in dilute form, cure it. This important discovery became the first principle of homeopathy, the theory of "like cures like."

Another law of homeopathy dictates its medicines be given in a minimum dose. Part of Hahnemann's frustration with allopathic medicine (a term devised by homeopathic practitioners to describe conventional medicine), was allopathic drugs, which caused nasty reactions. To avoid this, he diluted his remedies to a point where no side effects were felt, but a cure was still possible. In fact, the more he diluted his remedies, the more potent they became. He believed the vigorous shaking, or successions, used to prepare his medicines, potentized them.

In classical homeopathy, the law of the single remedy demands its medicines be given one at a time based on current symptoms. Because the patient and disease are each seen as fluid and ever-changing, the remedy is altered as the symptom picture changes. In homeopathy, the focal point is the patient, not the illness. This concept requires the homeopathic practitioner carefully documents as many details of his patient's health as possible: physical symptoms, emotional and mental balance, food cravings and aversions, sleeping habits and other, sometimes seemingly bizarre, observations.

These symptoms are then painstakingly matched to one of over 2000 remedies made from plants, minerals and animal matter at an appropriate minimal dose. The closer the match, the more effective the remedy will be. This invariably takes much more time than your typical doctor visit.

## *Herbal And Homeopathic Remedies Provide Natural Solutions*

Homeopathic practitioners believe the natural state of a human being is one of health and our bodies possess the ability to heal themselves. When symptoms are suppressed, as is often the case in allopathic medicine (and sometimes natural medicine) the problem is buried instead of unearthed.

Symptoms like fever and inflammation are your body's attempts to heal itself. The heat of a fever helps destroy germs; the swelling and redness of inflammation indicate your immunity system is hard at work. Dismissing your body's signals not only ignores its desire to heal, but also leaves it ignorant when the next bacteria or virus attacks. Like yourself, your body learns by doing. By allowing your body to experience an illness without interference, you prime your immune system so it's ready for the next attack. This is why homeopathic remedies and herbs are so great—they support your body's natural healing abilities without taking over.

Many synthetic drugs have unpleasant and sometimes dangerous side effects. Instead of boosting your immunity, many medications cripple your body's defenses. In the case of antibiotics, the bugs have become smarter than the drug. Since the first report of antibiotic-resistant staph in Australia 30 years ago, bacteria have been fighting back at an alarming rate.[3] As antibiotic arsenals dry up, many physicians worry they'll be without medicines for serious conditions like pneumonia and meningitis.[4] That's where natural medicine comes in—safe effective treatments without long-term consequences.

We've been talking in generalities about natural medicine in this chapter. Now, I want to explore some conditions that are directly influenced by an imbalance of female hormones. For myself, PMS was a curse. You might be plagued with hot flashes and night sweats, common symptoms of menopause. Whatever your complaint, I have some specific suggestions for you to try. Wild yam, is of course, the focus of this book because of my great success in using it. However, I've also created a chart of other female-oriented herbs and their healing properties. Please refer to Appendix C: Herbal

Materia Medica, to discover some of the wonderful remedies available along your road to natural solutions. These herbs have been incredibly important to me along my journey of discovery. I know they can help you, too!

# Summary

- Natural medicine is centuries old.

- Herbal medicine is the art and science of studying plants for healing purposes.

- Over 5,000 plants have been studied for medicinal properties.

- Many drugs are made from, or based on plant compounds.

- Herbs support the body's healing process.

- Herbal preparations include teas, pills, creams, salves, ointments, creams, essential oils and tinctures.

- Herbal quality varies.

- Homeopathy is based on the principles that "like cures like", "minimum dose" and "single remedies."

- Your body wants to heal itself.

# Chapter 2

# HORMONES ARE US

JUST WHAT DOES WILD YAM have to do with hormones? Since in my experience wild yam has helped a wide range of female hormone conditions, I wanted to understand how my hormones worked. My previous understanding of hormones was limited, so I read everything I could find on the subject. You may have noticed signs that your hormones aren't functioning as they should–feeling grouchy or moody are hints. By discovering how hormones work in your body and regulate your menstrual cycle, you too can understand how wild yam and other medicinal plants may benefit hormonal problems.

Extreme hormonal fluctuation can disrupt your serenity, work, relationships and well-being each day of your life. Family members might suggest you see a psychotherapist for treatment of your crazy mood swings–laughing one minute and crying the next. Life becomes an emotional roller coaster for you and everyone around you! Many women have no logical explanation for these yo-yo emotions and other symptoms.

Most look to their gynecologists and other specialists for solutions, but often with few results. Maybe your doctor has prescribed medicine for you with uncomfortable side effects and minimal help. Some women you know (or you may do this yourself) look for instant solutions, such as taking antidepressant drugs to combat depression or going on diet pills to lose weight caused by water retention. However, drugs aren't curative! They just mask symptoms. As so many of us have found out, drugs can even aggravate our troubles.

## *PMS since age 13*

Jeanne is one of the many women who has shared her story with me. She told me she'd been suffering from PMS since she was 13 years old. Then six years ago, her doctor prescribed progesterone capsules for those "in my head symptoms." Finally she discovered wild yam cream. After using it for only a couple of days, her PMS, bloating and anxiety diminished.

# Hormones Aren't Child's Play

A woman's physiology is complex. Our hormones fluctuate greatly depending on where we are in our life–puberty, menstruation, pregnancy, breast feeding or menopause. Even within a month's time, your hormones jump up and down like the blips on an EKG. This is normal. Without this hormonal ebb and flow, your special female qualities would be lost. The challenge women face is the discomfort from hormones that jump around too much. Many people call this "hormonal imbalance."

During my many discussions with women, doctors and experts in the medical field, I've been told that over 75 percent of women at some time in their lives experience symptoms related to hormonal imbalance–sometimes they're not even aware the cause is hormonal. Have you ever been irritable, bloated, depressed, craved sugar so bad you ate spoonfuls from the bag or had menstrual cramps? Did you know these symptoms could be due to wild hormones? Perhaps you've experienced the hot flashes, insomnia, anxiety, and night sweats related to menopause. Are you concerned about bone loss in your post-menopausal years? Overly fluctuating hormones could be a contributing cause.

When you acknowledge the cause of your "woman problems" may be hormonal, you can take intelligent and effective steps to shift your body back into balance. You can make your system whole and healthy again with natural solutions. I did! During my healing journey, I learned how hormones work in a woman's body. Along the way, I discovered a safe road that corrected hormone problems using natural therapies.

# What Are Hormones?

The word "hormone" comes from the Greek word meaning to excite or to stir up. Immediately, I think of the sex hormones! The word sex brings up feelings of passion and excitement. How appropriate that hormone means to stir-up. When my hormones "stir-up," I effectively "excite" everyone around me! Your hormones are imperative to your health. These chemical substances direct, regulate, and coordinate the activities of your entire system. It's true that hormones manage basic sex drives and the reproductive system, but they also promote growth, control body temperature, maintain energy, repair tissues as well as aid in water and salt metabolism.

For example, estrogen, a steroid hormone, is made largely by your ovaries. This sex hormone is responsible for growth, development, maintenance and function of your sex organs. Estrogen is what gives you feminine characteristics like soft skin and an hourglass figure. In the next chapter, I will address this and another incredibly important sex hormone, progesterone, in more detail. For right now, you need to understand that estrogen and progesterone regulate the reproductive cycle and determine how you experience adolescence, menopause and all the years in between and beyond. Hormones have a powerful influence and effect on every cell in your body. To further your understanding, let's take a closer look at the function of hormones, where they come from and how they get where they are supposed to be going.

# Where Do Hormones Come From?

Hormones are produced and secreted by the endocrine glands–thyroid, pancreas, pineal, thymus, ovaries, testes, adrenals and parathyroid–into the bloodstream to evoke a response in another part of your body. This very large and important family of glands is your endocrine system. Your endocrine glands grab amino acids, cholesterol and other ingredients from your body, mix them up and make hormones. Each gland has its own job to do, but they all work together, too, so your body will run smoothly.

# Who's In Charge Of The Endocrine System?

The conductor of the endocrine system is the anterior pituitary gland, nestled at the base of your brain. It's this gland that operates the feedback mechanism that controls where hormones are going and when they need to be shut off. This system works somewhat like a small computer in your body, sending and receiving messages. The big boss is the hypothalamus which sends special hormones called releasing factors to the pituitary, instructing it how to manage the other endocrine glands.

As you've probably guessed, the endocrine system is a busy place. It reminds me of those cloverleaf highways in Los Angeles where cars are zipping all over the place. Your hormones are like those cars, and the exits are the different cells and tissues in your body. LA drivers get to their destinations by reading street signs. Your hormones work the same way. Not all hormones effect all cells in your body. When cruising through your bloodstream, hormones depend on specific hormone receptors–"street signs"–on designated cells to direct them.

Once a particular hormone has found its "target" cell, then a cascade of chemical reactions kicks that cell into action. Without a receptor to receive the hormone, nothing can happen. You can also think of receptors as a lock and the hormone as the key that opens that lock. Once a hormone "opens" a cell up, depending on the hormone and the type of cell it fits, any number of things can happen. That cell might make more hormones, it could produce protein or cause a muscle cell to contract.

Throughout your body there are receptor cells for estrogen and progesterone. For example, both estrogen and progesterone receptors reside in your breasts. Estrogen makes your breasts firm and full, while progesterone has the opposite effect and leaves them soft and mushier. If you have PMS, your estrogen levels most likely overshoot during the last half of your cycle and your progesterone falls too low. Have ever wondered why you have breast tenderness or swelling a few weeks before your period? It could be that you have too much estrogen clogging up the receptors on your breast cells creating full, firm, swollen breasts.

Synthetic progesterone (called progestogen) won't help your aching breasts. While man-made progesterone is similar in structure to your own natural source, it's not close enough to reduce symptoms. Your body does not have receptors to fully recognize synthetic hormones, therefore your symptoms continue and may even worsen with these drugs.

Under normal conditions, there is a harmonious balance between the endocrine glands, nervous system, and the response of the receptor cells. If a gland or some related part of your body isn't working right, a hormonal deficiency or excess can occur, causing what some call an imbalance. Stress or improper diet, for example, can adversely affect your glands, disrupt your feedback mechanism and upset hormonal secretions.

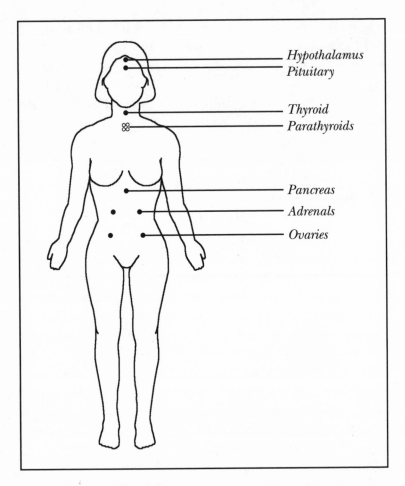

# A Personal Introduction
# To The Endocrine System

I've told you how the endocrine system generally works. Let me personally introduce you to each of the glands and organs and tell you a little more about them and their hormones.

## *The hypothalamus*

The hypothalamus gland plays a major role in regulating your menstrual cycle and the production of female hormones.

Located in the brain, it activates messages sent to the endocrine system and is linked to your nervous system controlling countless bodily functions like body temperature, thirst and hunger. The hypothalamus is sensitive to physical and emotional stress which can affect its ability to send signals to the anterior pituitary. These upsets can alter what the hypothalamus tells the pituitary, and thus the rest of the endocrine system. The ultimate result may be topsy-turvy hormones and an irregular menstrual cycle.

## *The pituitary*

The pituitary gland is a small body joined to the hypothalamus at the base of your brain. The pituitary is actually divided into two separate glands–the anterior pituitary and the posterior pituitary. The anterior pituitary gland supplies a special brand of hormones that control your endocrine glands and regulate your menstrual cycle. The anterior pituitary also releases its own set of hormones, namely prolactin, the breast feeding hormone, and growth hormone.

The posterior pituitary, a neighbor but unrelated to the anterior pituitary, is responsible for two hormones–antidiuretic hormone (ADH) and oxytocin. ADH helps you maintain arterial blood pressure, for example, during blood loss, by retrieving water from your kidneys. Oxytocin contracts the uterus during childbirth and causes milk let-down during breast feeding.

## *The pineal*

Your pineal gland is a member of the endocrine system, but isn't really a gland. Nerve messages tell the pineal when to release its hormone, melatonin. Your pineal gland and melatonin are thought to keep your biological clock ticking. Temperature, light and emotions command the pineal gland regulating your sleep, mood, immunity, aging and your menstrual cycle.

## The adrenals

An adrenal gland sits on top of each kidney. Each adrenal consists of two parts–the cortex and the medulla. All adrenal hormones are ruled by adrenocorticotrophic hormone (ACTH) from the anterior pituitary. The adrenal cortex is the outer part of the gland responsible for making and secreting three kinds of steroid hormones. The first kind, called mineralocorticoids, includes aldosterone which keeps your blood pressure normal by balancing sodium, potassium and fluid levels.

Your doctor might have prescribed cortisone for you at some time. This popular drug is very much like the glucocorticoid hormones, cortisol and corticosterone, also made by your adrenal cortex. Besides reducing inflammation, these hormones regulate blood pressure, support normal muscle function, promote protein breakdown, distribute body fat and increase blood sugar as needed. Your adrenal cortex also manufactures small amounts of the sex hormone estrogen, and the male hormones testosterone and dehydroepiandrosterone (DHEA).

The medulla is in the inner part of the adrenal gland that acts more like it's a part of your nervous system than your endocrine system. The medulla's hormones, epinephrine (also called adrenaline) and norepinephrine, are controlled by the sympathetic nervous system when you're scared or mad. When these hormones are released, your heart pounds, your blood pressure soars and you're ready to fight!

## The thyroid and parathyroid

Your windpipe is straddled by the two lobes of your thyroid gland, and snuggled in their underbelly are four tiny parathyroid glands. The thyroid gland produces the hormones thyroxine and triiodothyronine–essential for growth, body temperature, regulation of proteins, fats, and the breakdown of carbohydrates needed for energy. Calcitonin, a blood calcium-lowering hormone, is also released by the thyroid and parathyroid. Your parathyroids ("para" means beside) emit parathormone (PTH) that controls phosphate and calcium metabolism for keeping your bones and nerves healthy. Thyrotrophin from the anterior pituitary keeps your thyroid hormones in check.

## *The thymus*

Squeezed behind your breast bone and just below the thyroid is an irregularly shaped member of both your endocrine and immune systems–the thymus gland. Your thymus grows until you're a teenager, then shrinks with age as fat fills in for the lost lymphatic tissue. Your thymus hormones are thymosin, thymopoeitin and serum thymic factor. They supervise several immune operations, particularly those that protect you from yeast, fungi, parasites, viruses, cancer and allergies.

## *The pancreas*

The long slender pancreas lurks behind your stomach. You're probably most familiar with the insulin and glucagon it makes, released by the islets of langerhans. These opposing hormones cooperate to keep your blood sugar even. Glucagon works together with epinephrine, growth hormone and glucocorticoids to prevent your blood glucose from dipping too low. High blood sugar calls your insulin into action, making sure glucose is passed from your blood into your muscles and body fat.

Your pancreas is a multi-talented organ. Did you know that without your pancreas, you wouldn't digest your food very well? Besides its endocrine duties, the acini cells of your pancreas make and spill 2 1/2 pints of digestive enzyme-containing juice each day–amylase for starch, lipase for fat and protease for protein–into your small intestine.

## *The ovaries*

The ovaries are a pair of small almond-size female endocrine glands that are connected to either side of the uterus via fallopian tubes. Your ovaries take turns releasing one egg per month during ovulation. The ovaries produce estrogen and progesterone, hormones that make you a woman with your menstrual cycle, large breasts and hips, and soft skin. Pregnancy also depends on these hormones, as well as breast feeding. During pregnancy, the placenta also produces progesterone and estrogen, taking over from your ovaries.

## *The testes*

The testes are a man's source of the male sex hormone, testosterone.

# Defining Womanhood– The Menstrual Cycle

Each month a woman experiences a menstrual cycle. That means for the average woman who menstruates for 40 years, she has 500 periods over her lifetime. The cyclical process of menstruation is a delicate and complex one–it's no wonder women experience so many physical and emotional changes throughout the month. You might find you feel really good one week a month. The rest of the month you may experience changes similar to the Dow Jones: Up-and-down-and-up-and-down.

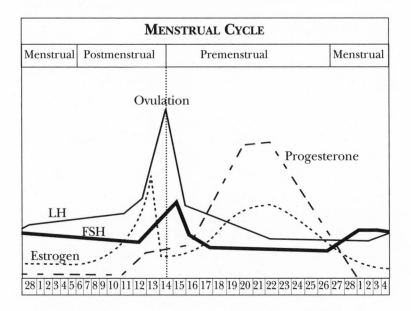

| MENSTRUAL CYCLE | | | |
|---|---|---|---|
| Menstrual | Postmenstrual | Premenstrual | Menstrual |

## THE FOUR PHASES OF YOUR MENSTRUAL CYCLE

**Phase 1: Menstruation**
Days 1-5: Menstruation occurs, estrogen levels are low and then begin to rise. Pituitary secretes FSH.

**Phase 2: The follicular or estrogenic phase**
Days 6-8: Estrogen levels continue to rise, egg-producing follicle grows.

Days 9-12: Fertile-type mucous is produced by the cervix to help sperm find the egg. Pituitary begins secreting LH.

**Phase 3: Ovulation**
Days 13-16: Ovulation occurs and LH begins to fall. Estrogen peaks and then decreases slightly. High estrogen levels turn FSH off. Basal body temperature dips then rises.

**Phase 4: The luteal or progesterone phase**
Days 17-20: Progesterone begins to rise. Estrogen rises again slightly. Egg travels toward uterus.

Days 21-24: Estrogen and progesterone levels peak then begin to fall. FSH and LH also on the decline.

Days 25-28: Body prepares to eliminate uterine lining–menstruation.

If one segment of your hormonal process is off, your entire cycle may suffer. Often you don't even realize why you're feeling tired, or in pain, or suffering unusual menstrual or ovulatory symptoms. During your menstrual cycle, estrogen, progesterone and other hormones are continuously on the move. Your well-being depends on a proper balance between estrogen and progesterone, as well as appropriate levels of FSH and LH. Once I understood these changes, I was able to identify that my hormonal problems were manifesting as PMS. Let me explain it to you.

Your body prepares and expects a baby every month of your menstruating years. It does this by lining your uterus with a rich, spongy bed of blood vessels, glands, and cells–not unlike a soft cuddly crib. When that doesn't happen, menstruation cleans out the uterus and tries again. While the uterine crib is being made-up, your ovaries harvest several eggs and then pop out the best one. If your egg doesn't meet a sperm, your womb sheds its lining–strips the bed so to speak–and starts anew.

The day you begin to bleed is day one of your cycle, which averages 28 days (although most women have normal cycles ranging from 20 to 40 days). A simple way of visualizing how your hormonal process works and how that correlates with the journey of the egg, is to divide your cycle into four phases.

It's your hypothalamus, the queen bee of the endocrine system, that kicks menstruation, the first phase, into gear. With messengers called follicle-stimulating hormone-releasing factor (FSH-RF) and lut-einizing hormone-releasing factor (LH-RF), the hypothalamus notifies the pituitary, the middle manager in female reproduction, to make its own hormones–follicle stimulating hormone (FSH) and luteinizing hormone (LH). These pituitary hormones are easy to remember because their names describe exactly what they do. FSH stimulates the follicles or pre-egg pouches in your ovaries. LH forms luteal tissue, that is the corpus luteum or remains of the mature egg follicle.

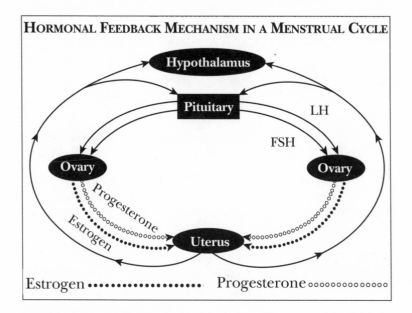

**HORMONAL FEEDBACK MECHANISM IN A MENSTRUAL CYCLE**

Hypothalamus

Pituitary

LH

FSH

Ovary          Ovary

Progesterone

Estrogen

Uterus

Estrogen •••••••••••••••••••  Progesterone ○○○○○○○○○○○○○○

---

*Hypothalamus secretes:*
  1) Follicle stimulating hormone-releasing factor (FSH-RF).
  2) Luteinizing hormone-releasing factor (LH-RF).

*Pituitary secretes:*
  1) Follicle stimulating hormone (FSH).
  2) Luteinizing hormone (LH).

*Ovaries*
  1) FSH stimulates the development of follicles.
  2) Follicle secretes estrogen.
  3) LH stimulates ovulation.
  4) Corpus luteum (left after follicle releases egg) secretes
     progesterone.

*Uterus*
  1) Estrogen stimulates a spongy bed-like endometrium to form
     inside the uterus during first half of cycle.
  2) Progesterone maintains uterine lining during second half
     of cycle.

Once you stop bleeding (around day 5 or 6–everyone is different) then the follicular or estrogenic phase starts. As you can see, each phase is named according to what hormone (in this case estrogen) or event (follicle maturation) dominates. Your pituitary sends FSH down to your ovaries so the follicles in your ovaries can grow up and become eggs.

Each one of us is born with as many as 400,000 follicles that last for life. This is unlike men who produce a fresh batch of sperm every few months until they die. Not all of these follicles get a chance at the big time, namely ovulation. Some mature, but then dissolve. Others merely deteriorate with age. But as I'll explain later, when your follicles run out, then menopause is just over the hill.

It's the maturing follicle within your ovary that secretes estrogen and gets the spongy uterine lining called the endometrium ready–the crib for the fetus we mentioned earlier. I like to think of estrogen as the maid of the reproductive system. She's there during the first half of your cycle, bustling around getting the nursery set for a fertilized egg. (Of course, estrogen has other effects on your body, but we're concentrating on the menstrual cycle right now.) Estrogen continues to rise during this time and then peaks. When estrogen levels are high enough, FSH secretion is turned off and your pituitary sends out LH instead–around day 10.

LH causes ovulation, the release of an egg from one of your ovaries; your ovaries usually take turns ovulating every other month. Ovulation occurs at the midpoint or third phase of your cycle, usually around day 14. Once it escapes from the ovary, your egg begins its journey down the fallopian tube where it will be fertilized if sperm reach it. This is called conception. You might feel a slight twinge or mild crampy sensation in your abdomen during ovulation. Doctors call this *mittelschmerz* which literally means "middle pain" in German. Some women feel nothing.

If you practice natural family planning and chart your basal body temperature (BBT) upon waking every morning, you may notice a dip in temperature the day before ovulation, and a rise of about 4/10 of a degree Fahrenheit the day after ovulation, caused by upward surge of progesterone. However, temperature can increase a day or two before ovulation too. This is why you can't depend on BBT as a reliable form of birth control. This temperature remains elevated if you are pregnant, and will drop just before menstruation begins if you're not.

The luteal phase begins the second half of your cycle (and fourth phase). Once the egg has left your ovary, the pituitary begins to secrete increased quantities of luteotropic hormone (LTH). LTH acts on the egg's remains left in your ovary (called the ruptured egg follicle) and converts it into the corpus luteum. The corpus luteum, Latin for yellow body, begins to produce more progesterone and slightly less estrogen. Progesterone is like a nanny who keeps your uterus spongy and ready for baby to appear.

Even though estrogen is the boss during the first half of your cycle, and progesterone during the second, it's not an all-or-nothing situation. Estrogen levels are still relatively high after ovulation. In fact, both of these hormones are vital to keep a pregnancy going. Estrogen takes care of your womb by enhancing uterine muscles, making sure there's lots of blood and preparing your breasts for nursing. Progesterone, on the other hand, relaxes your womb so you don't go into labor prematurely. It also calms your bowels and stomach so you absorb more nutrients, important for a growing fetus.

As I've said before, these two hormones work in opposite but cooperative ways. It's like the perfect partnership where each member knows her place and picks up where the other leaves off.

These higher progesterone levels inhibit pituitary production of LTH. As LTH falls off, the corpus luteum breaks down. Without sufficient amounts of progesterone to maintain the uterine lining, the corpus luteum (now called corpus albicans or white body) dries up and stops making hormones. The egg joins the soon-to-be menstrual fluids in your uterus. Then, your menstrual cycle occurs all over again.

## What If There's A Baby?

If conception occurs, the placenta eventually takes over progesterone and estrogen production from the corpus luteum. The placenta also makes another hormone called human chorionic gonadotropin (HCG). This is what pregnancy tests measure. HCG increases estrogen and progesterone production to maintain the pregnancy. Both FSH and LH levels decrease at this point.

## Harmonious Hormones

The rise and fall of estrogen and progesterone during your menstrual cycle and years beyond is the foundation for health and well-being. Once I figured out how hormones worked in general and the ins-and-outs of my period, the next step in my journey of discovery was uncovering more information about the specific functions of estrogen and progesterone. I wanted to learn how I could achieve a harmonious hormonal balance and good health.

Let's talk about these hormones in the next chapter. Many women's health conditions are related to an imbalance of these hormones. Understanding the basic endocrine system, menstrual cycle and hormonal process is one more mile on the road to discovering natural hormonal solutions for your health care. You can do this and still remain free of drug side effects and stay healthy. Hormones truly are us!

## *Hormoans!*

*I was sick and tried of being sick and tired.*
*I was desperate.*
*I was on an emotional roller coaster.*
*My breasts were so big they felt like grapefruit filled with*
*water weight.*
*I felt like a balloon ready to pop.*
*I was overwhelmed by a dark and painful depression.*
*I was a walking misery.*
*My mind was fuzzy.*
*What was the cause of these effects?*
*Hormoans!*
*I had pain all over my body, it seemed.*
*I was exhausted and stressed.*
*The pain and exhaustion were staggering.*
*Even when I woke up, I was so tired I couldn't get out*
*of bed.*
*What was going on with my body?*
*Did I have a virus or infection?*
*Did I have cancer?*
*Thyroid problems?*
*Heart disease?*
*Why was my skin dry and flaky?*
*Was this just part of getting older?*
*Are you supposed to feel worse in your 30s?*
*Wasn't I too young to feel like this?*
*What was the cause of this?*
*Hormoans!*

*I never knew when this state would come over me.*
*I just knew it wasn't normal.*
*I had to do something.*
*I needed to feel good again.*
*I wanted my old body back.*
*The last time I felt really good was before puberty.*
*That was before my hormones stirred-up my life.*

*There must be a solution!*
*Who had the answers?*
*Where could I turn?*
*What could I do?*
*My doctors fed me pills, but I felt sicker.*
*Maybe Mother Nature had the answer to my questions.*
*I, like Mother Nature, am a wise woman.*
*The answers to my questions had to be . . .*
*Hormoans!*

I wrote this in my journal during the beginning of my search for natural solutions. ~MB

# Summary

* Hormones direct, regulate and coordinate activities in your body.

* Hormones attach to specific receptors on certain cells and organs throughout your body.

* The endocrine system is made up of several glands with different functions in your body.

* Hormones are made by endocrine glands (estrogen and progesterone are just two of many hormones).

* Hormones are controlled through a feedback mechanism.

* Progesterone and estrogen have opposing effects on your body.

* A balance between progesterone and estrogen is necessary for health and well-being.

- Your menstrual cycle can be divided into four phases.

- Progesterone and estrogen naturally rise and fall during your menstrual cycle.

# Chapter 3

# THE BALANCING HORMONES: PROGESTERONE & ESTROGEN

MANY WOMEN DON'T REALIZE it, but there is a continuous struggle going on in their bodies! It is fought between two hormones striving to balance each other. These hormones, progesterone and estrogen, can be the best of friends or the worst of enemies. If your body is healthy, these two powerful hormones stay in perfect balance, and you do not experience any symptoms or disorders—a truce, so to speak. Unfortunately, there are many women who have lost the war and whose hormones are out-of-sync. Thus, they suffer from the often debilitating physical, mental and emotional symptoms of this hormonal battle. Have you ever felt depressed? Moody? Do you have cysts in your breasts or irregular cycles? You will be surprised to learn the cause of your problem may be these hormones!

So who are the main contenders? Progesterone and estrogen—opposite personalities that are nevertheless attracted to one another. Like an old married couple, these sex hormones struggle with the difficulties of a close yet volatile union. You know how hard this kind of relationship is! If you're like I was, your hormones may be on the verge of a divorce. Until that happens, you don't know how this kind of imbalance affects your body.

To fully understand the relationship between progesterone and estrogen, I first researched their various functions. Only then, did I understand how important a healthy balance between the two was and how my "woman problems" could be resolved. I learned about estrogen replacement therapy (ERT) and the therapeutic use of synthetic hormones. I discovered, by talking with naturopathic doctors and other holistic practitioners, natural solutions that are available to resolve estrogen-progesterone imbalances.

# The Hormone Factory

I found it valuable to study how hormones are made in the body when I was reviewing the benefits of wild yam and natural progesterone. In my mind, each endocrine gland is like a tiny factory spewing out its particular brand of hormones. The process begins with cholesterol—that same fatty substance we try to avoid like the plague. I hate to tell you this, but while you're buying cholesterol-free margarine, your body is making tons of the stuff. Cholesterol has gotten a bad rap in the media. The truth is most cholesterol-rich foods also contain plenty of saturated fats. Cholesterol is found only in animal-based foods like lard, butter and thick juicy steaks. It's these foods which make you fat and clog your arteries. Without cholesterol, you would die. You need cholesterol to make cell membranes, lipoproteins, bile and, of course, sex hormones.

Once on the assembly line, cholesterol first transforms into pregnenolone. The next step in the conversion process is progesterone (depending on which biochemical conveyor belt you take) which can create DHEA, cortisol, cortisone, corticosterone, aldosterone, androstenedione, estrogens or testosterone. A healthy body is like a well run factory, producing only enough hormones to meet physiological demand. But

# BIOCHEMICAL PATHWAYS OF HORMONES

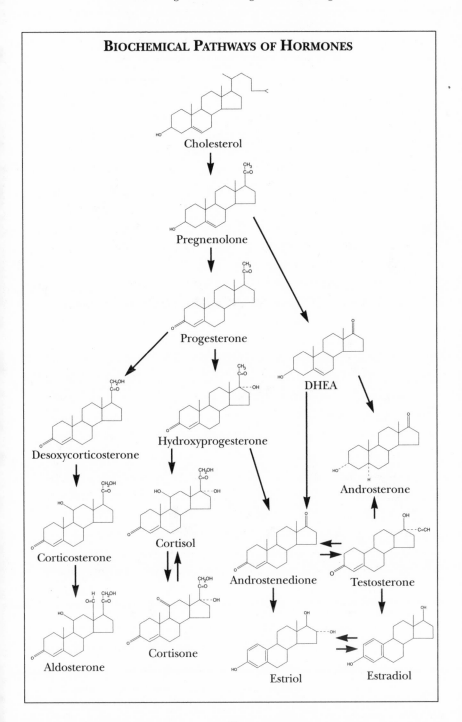

Cholesterol

Pregnenolone

Progesterone

DHEA

Desoxycorticosterone

Hydroxyprogesterone

Androsterone

Corticosterone

Cortisol

Androstenedione

Testosterone

Aldosterone

Cortisone

Estriol

Estradiol

when there's a problem in the system, then hormone orders get mixed up and you might manufacture too much or too little of a particular hormone.

# What Are Androgens?

There are three types of sex hormones in your body: progesterone, estrogen and androgens. Androgens are a group of male hormones. The strongest, and one you're probably most familiar with, is testosterone. Like estrogen and progesterone in women, testosterone gives men those typically male characteristics like a deep voice and facial hair, as well as maintaining their male reproductive organs.

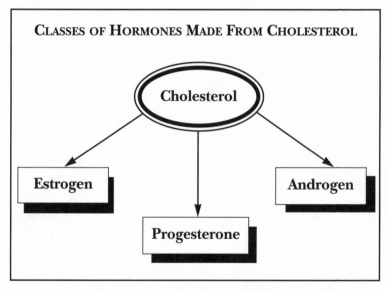

**CLASSES OF HORMONES MADE FROM CHOLESTEROL**

Cholesterol

Estrogen

Androgen

Progesterone

What you may not know is all women also have small amounts of these androgens, just like men have tiny quantities of estrogen. In fact, estrogens are formed from testosterone in a man, in his liver and other body tissues. A man's testes are the endocrine glands that produce most of his testosterone (and estrogen) as well as other androgens. Since you don't have testicles, then your adrenal glands make at least five different androgens in your body like androsterone, testosterone and dehydroepiandrosterone (DHEA). Your ovaries also make minute bits of testosterone.

Although the information I looked at is vague, women seem to need androgens for their tissue-building activity. Testosterone, for example, promotes protein synthesis which builds muscles. Why do you think athletes take anabolic (body building) androgen steroids? It's because they erect big, bulging muscles. Like the use of any synthetic hormone, problems can arise. Like progesterone and estrogen, your male and female hormones are in a relationship. When these girl and boy hormones aren't properly balanced in your body, it can turn into a battle of the sexes.

There's a condition called Stein-Leventhal Syndrome which occurs in some women—when male hormones are too high either from a tumor in the adrenal gland or ovary, or a problem with the communication system between the hypothalamus, pituitary and ovaries. If this happens, then beard-like hairs grow on your face and your period is very irregular or absent. As menopause approaches, the teeter-totter balance between your male and female hormones naturally tips ever so slightly toward your androgens and those same black stubby hairs may sprout on your chin.

I've always cherished being a woman, and once I found good health and a balance in my life and hormones, I loved my femininity even more. As I educated myself about hormones, I realized what a thin line separates male hormones and female hormones. Look at the picture below of testosterone and estrogen. There isn't much difference, is there? It really doesn't take much to convert one into the other in your body. Did you know both molecules are made from progesterone? It's truly amazing, even with all the potential hormonal problems we women have, how well Mother Nature keeps a handle on this intricate balance in our bodies.

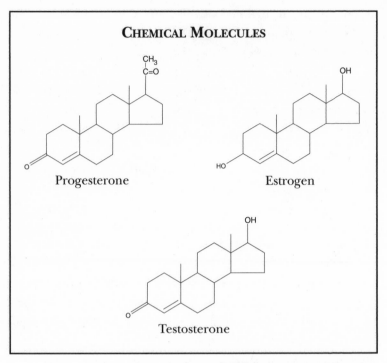

**CHEMICAL MOLECULES**

Progesterone

Estrogen

Testosterone

You may have heard about DHEA recently. Like the other sex hormones, your body can make DHEA from progesterone. (See Pathway Chart.) DHEA's job in your body has been fuzzy. We know it has slight androgenic properties. Researchers also thought this steroid hormone was a reservoir for your body to produce other hormones, like estrogen, progesterone and testosterone. However, it's becoming more apparent that DHEA has roles of its own. Its functions are still blurry, but according to Alan Gaby, M.D., author of *Preventing and Reversing Osteoporosis*, DHEA appears to affect your heart, body weight, nervous system, immunity, bones and other systems. (1) Recent medical studies on DHEA indicate it is therapeutically valuable for a wide range of medical conditions like cardiovascular disease, obesity, lowering cholesterol, depression, diabetes, cancer, Alzheimer's disease, immune system disorders and chronic fatigue syndrome.

# Defining "Progesterone"

Because there's so much confusion around what is prog-esterone, what is natural progesterone and what is synthetic progesterone, I'd like to begin this section by defining each of these terms.

- Progesterone: This is the female sex hormone made in your body.

- Natural progesterone: This is the term I'll use (and one you'll see in many books and articles) that refers to progesterone made from the wild yam, soybeans and sometimes animal sources. Natural progesterone is a regulated chemical called USP grade proges-terone. According to what many experts have told me, natural progesterone is identical in structure to the progesterone found in your body.

- Progestogen: This is a synthetic drug that has some progesterone-like effects. If you're taking proges-terone, chances are it's this most refined one. Because these progestogens possess a different molecular struc-ture than the progesterone found in your body, they act differently. Unlike the progesterone in your body which has anti-estrogen effects, progestogen has estro-gen-like actions (which can aggravate your PMS symp-toms) or androgen-like effects (which can "bring out the man in you" with unattractive facial hair) along with its progesterone-like qualities. Progestogens are usually made from natural progesterone. That is, the starting materials for progestogens are also wild yam and soybeans, but progestogens are more processed than natural progesterone.

The above three terms are what I'll be using throughout the book to refer to the various forms of progesterone. I also want to add these definitions to further clarify (or perhaps confuse) you.

- Progestional: This adjective merely describes any substance (usually progesterone or a progesterone-like drug) that helps maintain pregnancy in a woman.

- Progestins: This is a generic term for any substance, natural or synthetic, that exerts a progesterone-like effect. Progesterone, natural progesterone and progestogen all fit into this category.

# The Importance Of Progesterone

Progesterone is one of the most important sex hormones in your body. It is the middle-man between cholesterol and your steroid hormones that bring cortisol, aldosterone, estrogen and testosterone to life. Progesterone and estrogen have a love-hate relationship going on. Out of balance, they ruin your life. They can't live without one another, either. Most of progesterone's actions demand estrogen be present either before or during its biochemical actions.

Your body normally produces between 20 to 25 milligrams of progesterone a day from your ovaries, adrenals and body fat. Biochemist Raymond Peat, Ph.D., believes optimal levels of progesterone are absolutely essential to well-being. He states women must have sufficient amounts of vitamin A, cholesterol and a healthy thyroid for progesterone to be made. "Recent studies show progesterone prevents stress-induced coronary blood vessel spasms in aged hearts, probably explaining women's relative freedom from heart attacks, so long as they retain functioning ovaries."[2]

Because natural progesterone helps regulate hormone

---

### SOME ACTIONS OF PROGESTERONE

1. Governs the second half or luteal phase of your menstrual cycle.

2. Prepares for and maintains pregnancy.

3. Helps control abnormal menstrual bleeding by preventing your uterine lining from sloughing off prematurely.

4. Stimulates production of nutritional secretions in your fallopian tube to feed your fertilized egg prior to implantation.

5. Activates certain cells in your breast to assist in producing milk.

6. When pregnant, it is secreted in high doses by the placenta. If progesterone is low, miscarriage can occur.

7. It increases your body temperature around ovulation.

8. Builds new bone.

9. Elevates blood sugar.

10. Promotes breakdown of fats.

11. When progesterone levels are high, you might feel depressed.[3]

---

levels, it can be beneficial for the symptoms of menopause and PMS, and menstrual cramps. It's also been used to treat inflammatory conditions such as rheumatoid arthritis, as well as endometriosis, irregular uterine bleeding, osteoporosis, amenorrhea and threatened miscarriage. Uterine and endometrial cancers threaten you when you take synthetic estrogen therapy alone. This risk is less likely when progesterone is added to an estrogen regimen or used alone.

# The Importance Of Estrogen

Estrogen is one class of hormones produced by the ovaries, adrenal glands, male testicles, and the placenta. Estrogen is also produced in your fat cells during your childbearing years. After menopause, it is mostly produced by your adrenal glands. There are three hormones referred to as estrogens: Estrone (E1), Estradiol (E2) and Estriol (E3).

Quick Facts:

- Estrone (E1) is a weak form of estrogen made from estradiol and the male hormone androstenedione.
- Estradiol (E2) is the primary and most potent form of human estrogen secreted by your ovaries.
- Estriol (E3) is the weakest form, found in large amounts in your urine. Estrone makes most of the estriol; estradiol makes a little bit. [4]

Estrogen in a healthy, normal balance benefits your blood vessels, increases good cholesterol levels, makes you happier, enhances your memory, may prevent heart disease, slows down bone loss, and encourages youthful skin. Jerilynn Prior, M.D., of the University of British Columbia in Vancouver, Canada, has conducted research that suggests estrogen does not actually rebuild new bone density, but only prevents further bone loss.[5] Yet, as you will discover, synthetic estrogen is not without risk.

---

### SOME ACTIONS OF ESTROGEN

1. During the first half of your cycle it rebuilds the lining of your womb.

2. It stimulates the production of special mucus by your cervix to assist sperm in fertilizing your egg.

3. Is responsible for breast development.

4. Enhances HDL ("good") cholesterol levels.

5. Retards bone loss.

6. Excessively high estrogen levels may contribute to fibrocystic breast disease, endometriosis, PMS mood swings, infertility and painful cramping periods.

7. Lowers blood sugar.

8. Promotes fat production.

9. Creates anxiety, when too high.[6]

---

# All Estrogen Is Not Created Equal

Like varieties of apples, we now know there are at least three different types of estrogens, all with different effects on your body. Because the word "estrogen" is often used to describe all types of estrogen, you may be confused as to the type you may need. Before I describe to you how estrogens are used during what's called ERT or estrogen replacement therapy, let me remind you that all three estrogens are vital for your health.

Estradiol, being the most powerful, is also the most important and influential estrogen in your body during your premenopausal years. Once you reach menopause, then estrone takes over. This is because estrone is derived from androstenedione, the male hormone secreted by both your ovaries and adrenal glands. It's your body fat that converts most of the androstenedione into estrone. I know being overweight isn't healthy. But during menopause, fat has its place. The fatter you are, the more estrogen (estrone) you're blessed with during the menopausal years. Estriol, the weakest and sparsest of the estrogens, exerts minimal effects on you.[7]

Now that I've explained how your body works under normal conditions, let's talk a little bit about using synthetic hormones. First off, many doctors prescribe estrogen therapy—that is synthetic estrogen without progesterone or progestogen to balance it. This treatment is often referred to as "unopposed estrogen". This is a big mistake because as you now know, progesterone and estrogen are friends that need one another for a well-rounded hormonal relationship.

Secondly, synthetic estrogen is made from the urine of pregnant mares and contains estradiol and estrone (as well as other estrogen-like compounds). It's these two strongest forms of estrogen, when used in high, drug amounts which can cause problems like uterine cancer and abnormal vaginal bleeding. What about the PMS you're trying to cure? Don't use estrogen treatment in oral contraceptives or as ERT. Synthetic estrogen often causes the very symptoms you're trying to avoid like depression, breast tenderness and headaches.

For years, European clinicians have used estriol instead of estradiol and estrone because this weaker estrogen not only appears to be non-cancerous, but may actually protect you against cancer. A study in the New England Journal of Medicine revealed elevated estriol levels in animals guard them against the tumor-inducing effects of estradiol and estrone.[8]

## Why These Two Fighting Hormones Are Really Friends

Dr. John R. Lee believes "One of the paradoxes in female hormone physiology is that estrogen and progesterone, though mutually antagonistic in some of their effects, each sensitizes receptor sites for the other. That is the presence of estrogen makes your body target tissues more sensitive to progesterone, and the presence of progesterone does the same for estrogen."[9] The theory is progesterone blocks the action of estrogen on its receptors protecting you from too many of estrogen's effects on your body. Mother Nature knows best. She'd never think of giving you unopposed estrogen without the balancing influence of progesterone.

## Why Estrogen And Progesterone Get Off Track

Progesterone and estrogen are involved in a continuous cycle of creation, metabolism and break down. While it's important that both your estrogen and progesterone are at appropriate levels in your body, it's also vital to have a balanced ratio between progesterone and estrogen. When either of these allies get off track, then your hormonal ratio also loses its balance. Let me give you a few examples of how this happens.

- Your estrogen levels can be normal with a reduced progesterone level.

- You can have excess estrogen but normal amounts of progesterone.

Once these hormones are out of balance, your emotional and physical equilibrium can be affected. Often, you may not even realize several common health disorders and conditions affecting you can be caused by or influenced by a progesterone to estrogen ratio that's faltering. Have you ever experienced mood swings or skin blemishes? Do you have hot flashes, insomnia or vaginal dryness? If you have experienced any of these symptoms, the cause of your problem may be hormonal imbalance.

Ann Louise Gittleman, best-selling author of *Supernutrition for Menopause,* describes loss of bone density, thinning hair, and increased facial hair as symptoms of low progesterone levels. She describes a condition called "unopposed estrogen dominance," resulting from an imbalance in the hormone levels that allow estrogen to take over. She says this condition can increase your risk of breast cancer, bone density loss, and hypothyroidism.[10]

Lita Lee, Ph.D., enzyme therapist and consultant, believes that estrogen is produced by many cells in the body, and any type of estrogen supplementation is potentially carcinogenic. She also says that some animal-based foods, like commercial meat, milk products and eggs, contain synthetic estrogen. Other foods, like wheat germ, yeast and yeast-containing foods such as beer and wine, and herbs, including dong quai and black cohosh, naturally exert an estrogen-like effect on your body. If you consume any of these estrogenic foods or herbs in excess, your body may be unintentionally assaulted with more estrogen than you need or can handle. Dr. Lita Lee states a healthy balanced ratio of estrogen to progesterone is ten to one and hormonal disorders occur when ratios are less than five to one.[11]

Although Dr. Lita Lee points to estrogen-like plants, also called phytoestrogens, as a source of elevated estrogen, I should point out that these plants don't just increase estrogens in your body. They have more of a balancing effect. So if your body's estrogens are too high (like in PMS), phytoestrogenic herbs temper your natural estrogen by occupying some of your estrogen receptor sites. Because the estrogen-like activity in plants is much lower than synthetic versions, you have less estrogen upsetting your hormonal apple cart. On the other hand, if you suffer from an estrogen-low condition like menopause, phytoestrogens supposedly supply you with a little extra plant estrogen boost.

# Super Liver To The Rescue

Although it might strike you as odd, the liver, your largest internal organ, is a key player in the hormone balancing game. Tucked underneath your rib cage on the upper right side of your abdomen, your liver sticks to a hectic schedule of storing and filtering your blood, producing bile for fat digestion, squirreling away vitamins and iron, as well as having a hand in almost every metabolic system in your body.

Your liver also handles estrogen and progesterone. As the major filtering system in your body, your liver ensures that you're not overloaded with poisons, drugs—or hormones. One way it does this is by converting your sex hormones into milder, less active forms and disposing of extra amounts through your urine. For example, estradiol is converted into estriol, the weaker sex hormone.

When your liver is not functioning properly or if you are deficient in nutrients required to fuel estrogen conversion, then the estradiol to estriol makeover is blocked.[12] Being a liver in today's world is like being Superwoman. Pollution, food additives, drugs, cigarette smoke, alcohol, junk food, pesticides and sundry other chemicals we meet every day, mean double duty for your liver.

Your liver has to sort through all these toxins while trying to keep you safe. While keeping the toxin assembly line going, your liver must also keep an eye on hormones passing through. I know when I have too much to do, I get overwhelmed and don't usually do a very good job on anything. Your liver is the same way. It has to be "Super Liver," working extra hard to discard and convert estrogen even when there's a backlog of toxins. The result is you end up with high blood levels of estrogen, hormonal imbalance and unpleasant symptoms.

When you eat a healthful diet high in fiber, and low in sugar and fat, fiber binds to toxins in your intestinal tract and sweeps them from your body. A poor diet lacks vitamins and minerals which hamper your liver's job. Even smoking adversely affects your liver, and ultimately your estrogen levels.[13]

# Comparing The Effects Of Estrogen Versus Progesterone

Estrogen and progesterone are at times like the relationship between wife and husband. Everything estrogen does, progesterone counteracts by doing the opposite. Does this sound like someone you know? Although opposite in nature, estrogen and progesterone's relationship works fine when each partner is even tempered. But when one member dominates, that's when the trouble begins. For instance, progesterone has a sedative effect, while estrogen is a stimulant. When unopposed estrogen is given, it can cause food cravings, nervousness, lower pain tolerance, insomnia, infertility, inflammation, increase headaches and aggravate hot flashes. When progesterone is given for high estrogen conditions like PMS, or administered along with estrogen for menopausal problems, it counteracts these side effects. Progesterone acts as an anti-inflammatory, antidiuretic and stress reliever.

Like a marriage counselor who thinks talking to the wife while ignoring the husband will cure marital problems, many doctors prescribe estrogen therapy without its balancing partner, progesterone. When unopposed estrogen therapy causes irregular vaginal bleeding, progesterone helps out. When estrogen makes you bloat up with water, progesterone assists by regulating water, sodium and potassium excretion by competing with aldosterone, another hormone that also manages these functions in your body.[14]

Progesterone raises your blood sugar, while insulin and estrogen lower it and promote fat storage. Balanced blood sugar protects you against the irritability and emotional ups-and-downs peculiar to low blood sugar. Progesterone and estriol may protect you against cancer and fibrocystic disease of the breasts. High estrogen levels, on the other hand, tend to promote some cancers and growth of cysts.

# Estrogen Replacement Therapy (ERT)

As you'll see from the following passage, synthetic hormones carry with them many side effects. So you may ask yourself, why were they developed in the first place? Well, natural hormones—both the ones you produce and natural progesterone made from the wild yam—tend to be quickly broken down by your digestive system. Synthetic forms, on the other hand, retain their effectiveness even when taken as a pill by mouth because they are not dissolved immediately by your gut.

Many myths have swarmed around estrogen replacement therapy (ERT). In the 1960's, it was touted as a miracle hormone that granted women their youth and ageless skin. A decade later, doctors began warning us ERT may cause endometrial cancer. During the 1980s, scientists speculated ERT was responsible for post-menopausal breast cancer. Today ERT is considered a cure-all by many. Several doctors suggest estrogen for just about all hormonal problems you may have. Has your doctor offered you hormones to relieve your PMS symptoms or for menopause-like hot flashes, night sweats, vaginal dryness, or to prevent osteoporosis?

For many years, treatment for menopausal women consisted primarily of ERT. The rationale behind using this hormone is it helps your body adjust to declining estrogen levels during menopause by increasing your blood levels of estradiol. Estrogenic drugs are also used in oral contraceptives, for the prevention of miscarriages and to treat abnormal vaginal bleeding.

What risks do you face with ERT? What are your other choices? I did not think there was another choice until I learned about the wild yam and natural progesterone. I've found wild yam can relieve these symptoms without the side effects caused by ERT. If you haven't heard about natural options, you really don't have much of a choice. You can decide to use ERT or do nothing.

# ERT Effects

No drug is a magic bullet. Anytime you take a drug, you're likely to experience unwanted effects in addition to its therapeutic actions. Cold medicines, for example, dry up your nose, but also make you feel drowsy. Every woman needs to be aware of the adverse effects of estrogen replacement therapy. ERT side effects can include: depression, headaches, loss of sex drive, mood swings, fatigue, irritability, sudden shortness of breath, nausea, hair loss, vomiting, cramps, breast tenderness or enlargement, changes in the amount of cervical secretion, vaginal yeast infection, lumps in your breast, jaundice (yellowing of the whites of your eyes), swelling or tenderness in your abdomen, a spotty darkening of the skin, skin rashes, dizziness, faintness, changes in vision, involuntary muscle spasms, increase or decrease in weight, possible changes in blood sugar and fluid retention. Water retention is of particular concern for women with asthma, epilepsy, migraines, heart disease, and kidney disease because it can aggravate these conditions.

More serious side effects can include thickening of the uterine lining, and possibly endometrial cancer. Women who use ERT after menopause are more likely to develop gallbladder problems requiring surgery than those who do not use estrogen. A recent study reported a two to three times greater risk of gallbladder disease among women who had taken ERT or oral contraceptives (as an estrogen source) post-menopause. Estrogen can also cause abnormal blood clotting and strokes, so if you have heart or circulation problems you may want to avoid it. Your blood pressure may increase while on ERT.[15]

Many doctors (and women) are so determined on washing away menopausal symptoms, and preventing heart disease and osteoporosis (conditions that tend to increase in women after menopause), that often they forget how lifestyle fits in. What I have oftened wondered is—what did women do before ERT? Why are we so scared about heart attacks and breaking bones? Is ERT the only way to go? ERT is not for me!

Genetics, of course, determines how susceptible you are to any disease. I like to think of this as your weak point. When some people get stressed out, they get a cold. Others might suffer from a stomach ache or depression. It all depends on where your body is the frailest. So if there are heart problems and osteoporosis happening in your family, you might want to find a physician who knows about natural hormonal solutions, diet and lifestyle, and can guide you safely toward health.

If you just want to keep your heart and bones as healthy as possible, take care of the diet, stress and exercise in your life. All of these things greatly influence whether you're going to be a heart or osteoporosis patient or not. The trick is to take action. I'll talk more about preventive steps you can take later in Chapters Six and Seven.

# Hormone Replacement Therapy (HRT)

Now, hormone replacement therapy (HRT), a combination of estrogen and progestogen, is in vogue. Many physicians are recommending this for women as a protection against osteoporosis. Progestogen is meant to balance the hormonal ratio I keep talking about. Unfortunately, the list of side effects for progestogen is almost as long as the one for synthetic estrogens. The adverse effects are depression, fatigue, breakthrough bleeding, bloating and fluid retention, weight gain or loss, increased appetite, headaches, breast tenderness, nervousness, exaggeration of PMS symptoms, suppression of ovulation, increase in LDL cholesterol levels, and suppression of progesterone levels. If you are taking synthetic hormones and notice any of these signs, consult with a health care practitioner.

# Natural Progesterone Can Help

As you've probably realized, the subject of natural progesterone is complicated. So it's not surprising that it has been reported to help relieve the following:

Physical Symptoms and Conditions—Migraines and other headaches, epilepsy, fainting spells, muscle pain and stiffness, asthma, infertility, dry skin, hoarseness, backache, flu and colds, joint pain, blurred vision, fibroids, bloating and breast tenderness, hot flashes, inflammatory conditions like arthritis and bronchitis, miscarriage, allergies, gas and constipation, hypoglycemia, dry hair, toxemia of pregnancy, upper respiratory infections, fatigue and gallbladder problems.

Emotional and Mental Conditions—Depression, mood swings, lethargy, poor memory, aggression, anger, irritability, frustration, panic, mental exhaustion.

# Natural Progesterone Versus Progestogen

Many women and their physicians aren't aware or don't believe safe alternatives to synthetic ERT or HRT exist. Some physicians are waiting for studies to be completed on the wild yam and other plants, or new drugs made from them, which could take years. Fortunately, some practitioners using natural hormonal alternatives can provide us with clinical evidence that these therapies are effective and really do work.

Synthetic hormones such as progestogen are most commonly prescribed as part of HRT. Many women do not react well to synthetic hormones, and experience myriad side effects. You may have experienced these yourself, like weight gain or breast tenderness. You may have taken these hormones under the brand names of Provera, Norlutate, and Amen. The unpleasant side effects of synthetic hormones force many women to discontinue using HRT during the first year. Fortunately, natural progesterone made from the wild yam does not usually have these side effects. It is therefore considered to be a safer option. In fact, natural progesterone seems to relieve as many hormonal and PMS symptoms as progestogens trigger.

COMPARISON OF NATURAL VS. SYNTHETIC PROGESTERONE

Synthetic Progesterone
(Norgestrel)

Natural Progesterone

Dr. John Lee believes that "In Western industrialized culture, pharmaceutical companies buy natural progesterone (derived from yams) and then chemically alter its molecular form to produce the various progestins, which, being not found in nature, are patentable and therefore more profitable. Most physicians are unaware their prescription progestins are made from progesterone (from yams)."[16]

One drawback of progestogen is that its chemical structure is different from the progesterone in your body. Progestogen also doesn't act like your own progesterone does. It can't convert into other steroid hormones. When choosing a hormone treatment, it is important to remember that progesterone is the primary building block for all other steroid hormones and this alone distinguishes natural progesterone from progestogen. Instead of binding to the progesterone receptors in your body, most of progestogen binds to androgen (male hormone) receptors. This means progestogen has mild male-inducing effects like increased facial hair. There are minimal, if any, side effects with natural progesterone.

# Natural Progesterone Is The Choice For PMS And Menopause

Natural progesterone is preferred over progestogen as a PMS treatment. Niels Lauersen, M.D., founder of the first PMS clinic in the United States, suggests in his book *PMS: Premenstrual Syndrome and You,* that when your doctor prescribes progesterone treatment, you should make sure he's talking about natural progesterone not a synthetic. Dr. Lauersen discovered only natural progesterone is effective in combating premenstrual syndrome. His experiences with progestogens are that they don't diminish PMS symptoms and may even increase them. However, a couple of his patients have found relief using Provera‰ (a brand of synthetic progesterone). Dr. Lauersen believes that, "When a woman is treated with synthetic progestogens, her body becomes confused and produces less natural progesterone."[17]

The side effects of natural progesterone were compared to progestogens in menopausal women. Joel Hargrove, M.D., of Vanderbilt University Medical Center in Tennesse, achieved a 90% success rate treating menopausal patients with oral doses of natural progesterone for PMS. In his study, Dr. Hargrove compared oral micronized progesterone (natural) to oral progestogen therapy. He found the progestogens to have side effects such as increase in facial hair, depression, fluid retention, and headaches.

Dr. Hargrove found natural progesterone can safely be ingested in 200 mg per dose equal to progesterone levels normally seen during the luteal phase of a woman's cycle cycle—with no side effects.[18] Dr. John Lee has had similar results using natural progesterone cream. However, his patients required five-to-eight times less natural progesterone because it was applied topically (on the skin).[19]

---

## FACTS YOU SHOULD KNOW

**Synthetic names of estrogen and progesterone**

| Brand name | Types of estrogen |
|---|---|
| ⌐Premarin | Conjugated equine estrogens (urine from pregnant mares) |
| ⌐Estrace | Micronized Estradiol |
| Estratab | Esterified estrogens |
| Ogen | Estropipate |
| Estinly | Ethinyl estradiol |
| Estrovis | Quinestrsol |

**Estrogen Vaginal Creams**

| | |
|---|---|
| Premain | Conjugated equine estrogens |
| Estrace | 17 beta-estradiol |
| Ogen | Estropipate |
| Ortho Dienestrol | Dienestrol |

**Progestogens (synthetic progesterone)**

| | |
|---|---|
| ⌐Provera | Medroxyprogesterone acetate |
| Curretab | Medroxyprogesterone acetate |
| Cyrin | Medroxyprogesterone acetate |
| Amen | Medroxyprogesterone acetate |
| Aygestin | Norethindrone acetate |
| Norlutate | Norethindrone acetate |
| Norlutin | Norethindrone |
| Megace | Megesterol acetate |
| Oveerette | Norgestrel |
| Micronor | Norethindrone |
| Nor-Q.D. | Norethindrone, micronized oral progesterone |

---

# Cancer Risks

Fear of cancer plagues most women in America today. Cancer evokes such fear in us because the cause is so vague, and there is no definitive cure. How do we prevent cancer? We can pinpoint some contributing factors to this disease: genetic predisposition, exposure to radiation, possibly viruses, poor diet, lack of exercise, as well as toxins from our food, water and the environment. Medical research indicates that excess levels of some hormones, like estradiol, may contribute to cancer risk. Other hormones, such as estriol, play a role in preventing cancer. Decades ago, researchers knew very high estrogen caused cancer. Fifty years ago, research showed progesterone was central to steroid production. During the 1950s, the author of *Steroid Hormones and Tumors,* Alexander Lipshutz, discovered estrogen to be the only hormone to be carcinogenic. His study showed rats given estrogen developed tumors like uterine fibroid and even uterine cancer. However, the rats' cancer went into remission when progesterone and pregnenolone (the precursor to progesterone) were given. Lipshutz concluded that progesterone helps solve the problem of excessive estrogen.[20] Estrogen contributes to the growth of some tumors, especially those in the breast. Breast cancer cells can produce and secrete estrogen, so high levels of estrogen, from supplementation or an imbalance, may encourage the growth of these cancers.

A very important theory explaining cancer prevention is the relationship between estriol and estradiol and progesterone hypothesis. Estradiol is associated with an increased risk of breast cancer. However, estriol seems to prevent this disease. Your body needs smaller amounts of estradiol compared to estriol or estrone because estradiol is 12 times more potent than estrone and 8-9 times stronger than estriol.

A formula developed 30 years ago by Dr. Henry Lemon called the "estrogen quotient" measures the ratio of estrone to estradiol. Dr. Lemon tested his formula on two groups of women with active breast cancer. One group was given 2.5 to 15 mg of estriol while the others were not treated. Of the women receiving estriol, 37 percent experienced a remission. He discovered the estriol levels of women with breast cancer were 30 to 60 percent less than women who did not have cancer. Cancer improved in patients partaking in the therapy, theorizes Lemon, because he boosted their estriol levels. This suggests women have a higher risk of cancer when their estriol is low in comparison to estradiol and estrone. It also suggests replacement therapy with estriol may be a cancer cure and lessen women's risk of getting cancer.[21]

Progesterone appears to guard women from cancer, too. One study reported that a progesterone deficiency in pre-menopausal women increases their chance of developing breast cancer 5.4 times and their risk of death from cancer tenfold.[22] Low levels of estriol and progesterone in a woman's urine are another indicator that she's at higher danger of breast cancer.

A 1995 study conducted by Harvard researchers confirmed that HRT during menopause does significantly increase your risk of breast cancer. Seventy-thousand women participating in the Nurses Health Study took both synthetic estrogen and progestogen. The study found that progestogen did not counteract the negative effects of the estrogen, but may actually have encouraged synthetic estrogen's cancer-causing action, raising the risk of breast cancer from 30 percent (with ERT alone) to 40 percent. The study did find, however, that if you stop using synthetic hormones, your cancer risk is the same as women who have never used HRT. That's good news![23]

However, even for a relatively well researched product like synthetic estrogen, the cancer connection isn't clear cut. Another study found that the long term risk of endometrial cancer or breast cancer increases with ERT, not just while a women is on the estrogen therapy but for many years after it is discontinued.[24] Women on estrogen for more than a year increase their risk of cancer (particularly endometrial) 4.5 to 13.9 times versus non-users. This hazard appears to be reduced if progestogen is added in sufficient amounts, and for long enough to the estrogen. There may also be a higher chance of developing breast cancer when postmenopausal women use ERT long term; however the results on this are inconclusive. These are just some of the reasons why women are looking for safer, more natural options to synthetic hormones.

## Does HRT Benefit The Heart?

Researchers and doctors still believe that the reduced risk of heart disease that HRT supposedly provides outweighs the increased risk of breast cancer. As your estrogen drops, your chance of heart problems rises. However, Dutch professor Jan Vandenbroucke, M.D., says for the past 20 years, scientists have questioned whether estrogen benefits the heart. Three situations have fueled this debate.

Results weren't good in studies where estrogen was given to men to see if it prevented recurrent heart problems. Also, birth control pills, which contain estrogen and progesterone, tend to promote vascular disease in young women. Lastly, Vandenbroucke reviewed a large study investigating the effect of estrogen on death from heart disease. He found that women who had heart problems before the investigation began were excluded from the final results. He speculates that the progestogens used in HRT cancels out estrogen's heart-benefits, if any. Estrogen does appear to lower blood fats, which play a role in heart disease. If this is so, says Vandenbroucke, "A more direct attack on lipids would seem logical."[25] Many holistic practitioners agree. Rather than relying on hormonal therapy to decrease blood lipids, it would be far safer to use diet, botanicals, exercise, quitting smoking and nutritional supplements to achieve this goal.

## It's Time To Start Making Decisions

Knowledge is power. With what I've taught you so far, I hope you feel stronger and more prepared to start making new decisions about your health care. You now understand how an imbalance between estrogen and progesterone can cause some of the most severe physical and emotional problems known to womankind. You may have identified the cause of your problems as hormonal.

I believe the best approach is to begin with the safest and simplest treatments. Now that you are aware of the risk potential of synthetic hormones and know about natural therapies to correct these imbalances, why would you want to use synthetic hormones? After all, when HRT begins clashing with your natural hormones, the battleground is a very special place—your body!

Besides wild yam and natural progesterone, make sure you're eating right and exercising regularly. These easy steps not only make you feel better, they'll reduce your risk of osteoporosis and heart disease. Your diet also influences your hormones. For example, Vitamin B deficiency may slash estrogen effects by interfering with its ability to bind to receptor sites. The typical American diet of fatty foods, as well as drinking alcohol affects the removal and recycling of estrogen.

If you find self-treatment with wild yam and lifestyle changes aren't working for you, then evolve to the next level of treatment and seek professional guidance from a qualified natural health practitioner. They can offer you medical supervision and expertise in the treatments you've already tried, as well as more complex therapies like homeopathy and acupuncture.

If you still don't get relief, you can then try semi-natural hormones like natural progesterone derived from the wild yam. If this doesn't help, you can then turn to synthetic hormones with the help of your doctor. While I certainly don't advocate using synthetic estrogen and progesterone indiscriminately, there is a place and time for these treatments when all else has failed.

I believe my gentle, slow approach allowed my body to decide what it needed before I took risks with synthetic hormones. I am not opposed to synthetic hormones. However, why should take them if I have other options to try first, that will work equally as well? I believe in choices and options. Come with me now on my next stop on my road of discovery—Chapter Four: Wild Yam, Wise Yam.

# Summary

- Abnormally high estrogen creates hormonal imbalances that cause many "woman problems".

- The liver converts estrogen into a milder form.

- When the liver isn't functioning well, it affects hormonal balance.

- There are at least three different types of estrogen.

- Estrogen replacement therapy has many side effects.

- Progestogen has many side effects.

- Hormone replacement therapy combines synthetic estrogen and progestogen.

- Natural progesterone is derived from plants like the wild yam.

- Natural progesterone and wild yam offer a safe alternative to synthetic hormone therapies.

- You have choices.

# Chapter 4

# WILD YAM, WISE YAM

DURING MY JOURNEY OF discovery, I began to understand the swampy terrain of hormones (explored in Chapter Two) and the push-me-pull-you relationship between estrogen and progesterone (investigated in Chapter Three). Once I knew how my body worked, I hunted for natural treatments that would steady my "stirred-up" hormones. Since I wasn't a candidate for ERT or even birth control pills, wild yam cream became my salvation. Still, I had many questions. How can wild yam cream help me? How does it work and how do you use it? Is it safe? What's the difference between wild yam cream, progestogen and natural progesterone cream?

## Are You Skeptical?
## Are You Suspicious?

When I first began my information expedition, I didn't believe wild yam cream or natural progesterone cream would really help me. Believing it could benefit me was as crazy as my life! Even though my meeting with natural progesterone expert Dr. John Lee was inspiring, I was still very doubtful. How could extracts from a wild yam plant help end my endless suffering?

Fortunately, I had many qualified natural medicine health professionals at my disposal while I was working on a book editing project, *The Alternative Medicine Yellow Pages*. I asked them all the same questions in an attempt to confirm what I learned from reading Dr. John R. Lee's work—What do you think of wild yam cream? Will it help my PMS? Can it relieve the symptoms of menopause? Does it work for women who have had a hysterectomy and want to avoid taking synthetic estrogen?—Since I know you probably have many of the same queries I did, I've listed my questions and the answers I received at the end of this chapter.

While I scouted around for explanations and eventually tried wild yam cream and other natural treatments, my skepticism gradually transformed into confidence. Wild yam cream changed my life! It restored my vitality, mental health, emotional stability and my physical well-being. Without it, I wouldn't have this story to tell. So if you're ready, let me continue my tale starting with the plant-hormone controversy.

# Do Plants Have Hormones?

One of the buzz words circling above natural health discussions is "phytohormones." If you recall from Chapter One, phyto means plant. So this word literally means "plant hormones". Many doctors and scientists dislike this label, because plants don't produce hormones, only animals do. What the term phytohormone attempts to convey is that some plants possess constituents that have hormone-like effects on your body. Whether or not your body can use these compounds to make real hormones is unlikely, though some experts suggest it may be possible. We just don't know for sure.

Phytohormones (for lack of a better word) are found in several plants, both herbs and food. Many natural medicine practitioners believe these substances work by competing with your hormones (like estrogen) for the same receptor sites in your body. Herbs with estrogen-like effects, like licorice and fennel, have a long history as female therapies. Unlike synthetic estrogen, these phytoestrogenic herbs balance your estrogen levels—whether they be too high or too low.

The theory goes like this. For syndromes where your estrogen runs amuck (like with PMS), the phytoestrogenic compounds, guessed to be about 1/400th as strong as synthetic estrogen, crowd out your body's own estrogen. This in effect diminishes estrogen's effects and your symptoms. If you don't have enough estrogen (as in menopause), then phytoestrogens supposedly offer you an estrogen-like effect. You can see how beneficial these phytoestrogenic plants would be if you're concerned about protecting yourself against cancer and other problems caused by synthetic estrogen.

## Soybeans Are Winners

Because these hormone-like substances appear in food as well as herbs, many women have unknowingly been proving the advantages of plant therapy for centuries. Soybeans and soy based foods like tofu and miso are rich in the estrogen-like isoflavonoids genistein and daidzein. These weak "phytohormones" possess about 1/1000th of the activity of estradiol.[1] One study suggested the reason Japanese women have fewer hot flashes and other menopausal symptoms is their love of soy foods.[2] Every menopausal woman should have a soybean shrine in her house! Tofu anyone?

Research shows women in Western cultures experience more hot flashes than societies who eat large amounts of soy foods. It is interesting that women in countries consuming nutritious diets full of whole grains, fresh fruits, vegetables, and an abundance of soy foods, also endure fewer hot flashes than the average American woman. If you live in Japan, Malaysia, or even Africa, you may never know a hot flash! The phytoestrogenic constituents in soy foods call a truce between your hormones.

---

### FIVE EASY SOY PIECES

Increase the soy and its beneficial phytoestrogens in your diet using these simple steps. (Soy is also high in protein.)

1. Use soy milk in place of cow's milk. There's plenty of wonderful tasting soy milk products on the market. Try a few, and pick your favorite.
2. Bake with soy flour. Substitute some soy flour for the flour you normally use when baking cookies, muffins or loaves. Only use about _ cup because soy flour has a strong taste.
3. Eat soy cheese. Like soy milk, there's lots of soy cheese brands available in your health food store. Taste a couple and the next time you make a grilled cheese sandwich, use soy cheese instead.
4. Add miso to soup. A tablespoon or two of miso enriches your home made soups and adds valuable nutrients. Miso is available in a variety of strengths and flavors.
5. Toss soy beans into everything. Soak and cook up a couple of cups of soy beans, then freeze them for later use. Add a handful or so of soy beans to casseroles, pasta salad or as a garnish to green salads. They're delicious and nutritious!

---

# More "Phytohormone" Sources

Exciting research on the chaste tree berry—*vitex agnus castus*—and its treatment of menstrual cycle disorders as well as PMS is one more example of a plant that realigns your deranged hormones. *Vitex* is believed to increase the production of lutenizing hormone and inhibit release of follicle stimulating hormone, which in turn helps increase your ratio of progesterone to estrogen. Clinical observations by 153 gynecologists on 551 of their patients demonstrated vitex reduced menstrual disorders and PMS complaints when taken over several cycles.[3]

Another study successfully treated patients whose menstrual cycles were lopsided with vitex agnus castus. The second half or luteal phase of these women's cycles was too short due to extremely high amounts of the hormone prolactin. After three months of a daily 20 milligram dose of *vitex*, prolactin levels fell. As a result, the women's luteal phase normalized and regular progesterone synthesis was restored.[4]

Mother Nature provides us with a whole medicine chest full of plants useful for treating female conditions. Most of the herbs help other ailments too. Some of these herbs are dandelion, cramp bark, black haw, black cohosh, red raspberry leaf, hops, nettle leaves, alfalfa and skullcap. See Appendix C for descriptions of these and other herbs you may like to try.

# The Wild Yam Connection

Let's clear up any misunderstandings you may have about yams—of which there are at least 150 species. The wild yam—*dioscorea*—is not the same kind of yam we traditionally eat with turkey on Thanksgiving. (You wouldn't want to eat *dioscorea*, it's way too bitter!) Sweet yams don't bear the same therapeutic benefits as the wild yam I'm talking about.

The benefits of dioscorea lie in its roots, just like the yams you eat. Wild yam grows in the wet woods of Mexico, Guatemala, China, and parts of the United States. People around the world, including Native Americans, have used the wild yam root to treat a variety of conditions such as bilious colic, gastrointestinal irritation, asthma and rheumatism. Women have welcomed wild yam for its ability to ease their menstrual cramps, morning sickness and afterbirth pains. Recently, research even points to wild yam as a possible cancer cure.[5]

What is not clear, is whether or not wild yam helps hormone-related ailments. Many people praise wild yam as a plant with progesterone-like qualities, yet several researchers and doctors say this is untrue. You'll hear some people suggest that taking wild yam will give your body the building blocks needed for producing other hormones, like DHEA and estrogen. Many experts say this is impossible. When I reached this stretch of my search, I realized I had one more medical mud puddle to trudge through. Let me take you by the hand and guide you through this very murky issue.

# Wild Yam Stirs Up The World

Wild yam's progesterone claim-to-fame began quite recently. It was sparked in the 1940s when medical pioneer Professor Russell Marker developed a chemical process to transform diosgenin, a constituent of wild yam, into progesterone and other hormones. This was a fantastic discovery, since up until that time, steroid hormones (then derived from animals) for treatments were very costly. Marker's methods were much cheaper and more efficient.

Professor Marker's adventure began in 1943 when he traveled to Mexico City in search of the wild yam. While residing there, he isolated diosgenin from *dioscorea mexicana,* one of over 150 species of wild yam. Marker's comprehensive research eventually led to the development of first contraceptive pill. His wild yam breakthrough absolutely changed the world for women. In 1973, 200 million drug prescriptions in the United States came from diosgenin.[6]

Unfortunately, once the Mexican government discovered the value of their wild yam crops, they increased the price of their diosgenin by 250 percent. Botanists and herbalists attempted to grow *dioscorea mexicana* in the United Stages and other countries, but without success. Since then, drug companies and herbal firms have turned to other wild yam species (which also contain diosgenin). A popular species in this country and others is *dioscorea villosa.* Today, most drug companies in the U.S. who make birth control pills and other steroid hormones use the cheapest starting materials they can, usually stigmasterol from soybeans or cholesterol from wool fat.[7] Still, 60 percent of all steroid drugs worldwide start with diosgenin from the wild yam.[8] These hormones relieve asthma, arthritis, eczema, high blood pressure, migraines and treat menopause symptoms, menstrual cramps and PMS.[9] Think how many times you may have used a medicine made from the wild yam, yet you didn't even realize it.

## Support For The Wild Yam

Over the centuries, wild yam has been used to treat a range of female conditions from morning sickness to menstrual cramps. The question remains—Does the wild yam retain hormone-like qualities? I don't know. In fact, while many medical experts point out there's no evidence that wild yam specifically affects female hormones, the truth is we really aren't sure. In my eyes, this means there's a remote possibility that wild yam does mediate the hormonal contenders in your body: estrogen and progesterone. Some researchers must think so too, because there are currently several studies being done on the wild yam in this important area. Also, it's stories like the following that have convinced me of the power of wild yam cream.

A 28 year old pre-med student had a full hysterectomy. She had a whole list of menopausal complaints. She was told by her doctors she must go on estrogen replacement therapy for the rest of her life. As a pre-med student, she was clearly informed and aware of the high risks and side effects of drugs. Following her own intuition, she (like thousands of women around the country) had been using wild yam cream or natural progesterone cream with fantastic results. Many times, women have told their doctors how wild yam cream relieved their symptoms when other things have failed to work.

# How Does The Wild Yam Work?

It's the steroidal sapogenins found in the wild yam roots, like diosgenin, yamogenin and others, that are used to manufacture progesterone, cortisone, DHEA and other steroid humans for medical use. The wild yams from Mexico have some of the highest sapogenin content—about 40 percent diosgenin and 60 percent other sapogenins.[10] These sapogenins are such terrific raw materials because their molecular structure is nearly identical to that of progesterone and other hormones.

Just because we can transform bits of plant into human hormones in the laboratory, it doesn't mean our bodies can do the same thing. Or can they? As with most herbs, there is no scientific evidence at this time proving the body can use diosgenin in any way to synthesize hormones. Silena Heron, N.D., a naturopathic physician and long time herbalist from Sedona, Arizona, says, "You can't take *dioscorea* and put it in the body and get progesterone out of it. What you get are precursors (building blocks), and your body decides whether it is going to make it into progesterone or other hormones." If you look at the following chart, you can see how similar diosgenin and progesterone are chemically. It wouldn't take much for your body to tinker with the diosgenin from wild yam and form the hormone progesterone.

It may be the wild yam's liver supporting ability that makes it so useful for various female conditions. Recall "Super Liver" and how important it is in breaking down hormones. So perhaps, wild yam affects your hormones indirectly by working on your liver. Regardless of the speculations and arguments about whether wild yam qualifies as a hormone regulator or not, I know it works .because women tell me so all the time.

Toni is a woman in her thirties. She was on the Pill for 25 years to keep her hormones in check.

---

### DERIVATION OF PROGESTERONE FROM DIOSGENIN

Diosgenin

Progesterone

---

When she finally stopped using birth control pills, she felt like her life was becoming a complete wreck. She was plagued with early menopausal symptoms and bled heavily for over three weeks. Toni was worried and very tired all the time. She didn't want the hysterectomy her doctor recommended to stop the bleeding. After trying several natural remedies with varying degrees of success, one of Toni's friends recommended a wild yam cream. Toni was so excited about the prospects of a natural product that could stop her bleeding, she began to use about 1/4 of a two ounce jar over the next four days. Around the fifth day, her bleeding stopped and her menopausal symptoms disappeared; her period became as regular as clockwork.

# Two Different Substances

There is a great deal of misunderstanding about wild yam and natural progesterone. I hope I've made it abundantly clear to you that they are two different substances. Natural progesterone is a term often used to describe progesterone made from the wild yam. Wild yam contains diosgenin, the raw materials to make progesterone in the laboratory. Wild yam does not contain progesterone itself. Recall from Chapter Three, progestogens (a class of progesterone-like synthetic hormones) are in a group all by themselves. If wild yam does alter the progesterone, estrogen and other hormones in your body, refer back to my explanation of how these hormones are made in Chapter Three. This will give you a clearer idea of the pathways of these hormones and how wild yam could theoretically work.

# The Food & Drug Administration Has Their Say

The Federal Food, Drug and Cosmetic Act as passed in 1938 regulates the use of all food and drug substances. In 1962, the act was amended to require all the drugs marketed in the United States after that year must be proven both safe and effective for their stated use. A new drug application requires research, not just testimonials or market success, as proof that it works. Unfortunately, testing a new substance—be it a drug or natural product like the wild yam—is so expensive and time-consuming that it's unlikely that any company will be willing to go through the process.

# Wild Yam Cream

While you can take wild yam root as a pill, tincture or tea, many companies are offering it in cream form as well.

## A PEEK INTO THE HISTORY BOOK
## ON HORMONE COSMETICS

Cosmetics containing hormones were first marketed in the 1930s. They came about totally by accident. The workers who were handling estrogen extracted from the urine of pregnant mares noticed their skin turning soft and more feminine looking—a side effect of the estrogen! As a result of this, in 1936, estrogen creams were introduced as a cosmetic product containing 10,000 IU of natural estrogen per ounce. These creams contained a mixture of two kinds of estrogen—estrone and estradiol. Thus, began the claims that estrogen was a miracle anti-wrinkle cream the world had been awaiting.

In 1954, the Food & Drug Administration (FDA) informed the cosmetic industry to limit the estrogen content of these products to a concentration of 20,000 IU of estrogen per month, even though some earlier concentrations containing more than 10,000 IU caused side-effects such as abnormal vaginal bleeding. The FDA stated that estrogen in concentrations up to 10,000 IU per ounce appeared safe for application to the skin. They recommended consumers not to exceed two ounces per month.

Today, most products contain 7,500 to 15,000 IU of estrogen per ounce. Current proposed FDA guidelines, based on one ounce quantities, still suggest using no more than two ounces per month. A standard two ounce cosmetic jar (how convenient!) might include 20,000 IU estrogen, one milligram of progesterone (.5 milligrams per one ounce) and up to .1 percent of pregnenolone acetate.

Both cosmetic and herbal companies have to be very careful about what they claim their products can do. If product labels, promotional material or advertising allege the herb or cosmetic has therapeutic actions, then in essence it's considered by the FDA to be a drug. Drugs have much stricter regulations to follow than cosmetics or herbs. The safety and efficacy of cosmetics containing hormones are currently being investigated by a government panel that reviews over-the-counter (not prescription) drug products including creams. Stay tuned for the results of this one!

Why is this? Does it work? Like most of the information on this herb, wild yam creams were created based on our current understanding of natural progesterone, which is made from the wild yam.

Dr. John Lee believes the transdermal (means passes through the skin) creams made with natural progesterone are eighty times more effective than the pill form.[11] Why? The pill must pass through the digestive system and the progesterone is broken down and eliminated too quickly to be effective. A cream bypasses your digestion by absorbing through your skin and into your blood stream. Some of the hormone also connects with specific receptor sites on your skin.

Dr. Lita Lee reveals that, "Natural progesterone cream is anti-aging to the whole body, and if you rub it on, your pores shrink. I've had people tell me that their moles disappeared." Christina Northrup, M.D., an obstetrician/gynecologist from Yarmouth, Maine, and author of *Women's Bodies, Women's Wisdom*, recommends using a cream containing natural progesterone cream made from the wild yam to treat migraine headaches. She recommends 1/2 teaspoon of cream applied to soft skin areas once a day as a preventive measure. For relieving a migraine already in progress, she suggests placing 1/4 teaspoon of progesterone oil under the tongue every 15 minutes.[12]

Raymond Peat, Ph.D., uses natural progesterone cream to treat a wide variety of conditions. He has cured suicidal depression, epileptic seizures and blindness from multiple sclerosis with three to four applications of progesterone cream a day. He has also treated menopause symptoms with good results.[13]

Although not scientifically studied, physician and patient anecdotes report miraculously positive results with natural progesterone creams containing wild yam and other herbs. In my experience, and from the stories I hear from women around the country, herbal creams with wild yam but containing no natural progesterone are helpful, too.

# The Most Commonly Asked Questions About Wild Yam And Natural Progesterone Creams

It was my thirst for knowledge and unending questions that propelled me along my quest for better health. You may have specific questions like I did. To make your journey less rocky than mine was, I've put together the following list of questions and answers. You'll notice from my answers that I often group natural progesterone and wild yam together. However, these are two different substances. Also, we know a lot more about natural progesterone than we do about the wild yam—we are still learning about the latter. My wild yam information is based on my experience and interviews I conducted with doctors and women who've tried wild yam creams. If I don't satisfy your curiosity here, talk to your doctor. Always consult with a qualified health practitioner if you're unable to remedy your medical problem.

## *So, what is wild yam cream?*

Wild yam body cream contains the wild yam extract in a highly concentrated solution. It is made from one of 150 wild yam species. *Dioscorea Villosa* is commonly used. Wild yam contains diosgenin, the starting material for the manufacturing of natural progesterone and many other steroid hormones.

## *How does wild yam cream differ from natural progesterone cream?*

They are two different substances. The wild yam's most active ingredient—diosgenin—is used to make progesterone in the laboratory. Natural progesterone is identical to the progesterone found in your body. While not proven and still hotly debated among health experts, it is theorized that the dios-

genin found in wild yam may be used to make steroid hormones in your body (if your body is able and chooses to).
Some say diosgenin has a progesterone-like effect on your
body, although there is no scientific evidence supporting this
claim. If this is true, the diosgenin is much weaker than your
own progesterone.

## Are all the wild yam creams or natural progesterone creams the same?

No. Each cream is different. The percentages and concentrations of wild yam cream or natural progesterone cream in a
two ounce jar varies, as do all the other ingredients. Natural
progesterone, USP pharmaceutical grade, is obtained only by
prescription for medicinal treatments in a standardized
amount. Cosmetic creams containing USP grade natural progesterone can be purchased over-the-counter.

## If the percentage of wild yam is equal in different creams, will they work equally well?

No. Equal percentages do not mean equal strength. The form
of the wild yam plant, either dry or liquid, and the quality and
species of the wild yam used can affect the actual strength.
Usually a higher percentage indicates higher potency, but not
always, because the actual concentration of diosgenin, wild
yam's active ingredient, can vary. Because natural progesterone is created in the laboratory, its strength can be controlled. The FDA proposes a maximum of one milligram of
natural progesterone per two ounce jar of cosmetic cream (.5
milligrams per one ounce) and up to .1 percent of pregnenolone acetate.

## How do you use a wild yam or natural progesterone cream?

The cream is applied to the soft fatty areas of your body like the breast, inner arm, inner thigh, wrist, and abdomen—rotating periodically to a different area. The amount used varies depending on the individual and condition being treated.

## Why use a cream, and how does it work?

A cream is easy to use. Hormones, like progesterone, tend to be broken down very quickly by your digestive system. One way of bypassing digestion is through your skin with a transdermal cream. The estrogen patch is a good example of this process. Progesterone receptor sites on your skin also benefit from a cream.

## Do I need a prescription for wild yam or natural progesterone cream?

No. Wild yam or natural progesterone cream in "cosmetic" form does not require a prescription. Pharmaceutical UPS grade natural progesterone in any strength, used any other way than cosmetically, is only available as a prescription from your doctor.

## How long will it take for me to see any direct benefits from the wild yam cream?

Many women I've talked to see immediate benefits—within a few hours or days. Others may see a difference within a few menstrual cycles. Women report their menopausal symptoms can be relieved within a few days. I found my physical symptoms of PMS like breast tenderness were relieved in a cycle or two. However, my depression took four months to disappear.

It's important to remember the results really depend on you and your unique biochemical make-up!

## Will wild yam cream help my hot flashes?

Yes, women have reported to me that it reduces hot flashes in a few days. For excessive hot flashes, experts recommend daily supplements of wild yam cream or natural progesterone cream, applied every 15 minutes during a hot flash. If hot flashes still persist after a few cycles, add a phytoestrogenic herb like licorice root taken by mouth to your daily regimen until the hot flashes have subsided. Stress, poor nutrition and physical illness may contribute to the onset of hot flashes and other symptoms. If you're not seeing results, consult with your doctor to see if there may be another medical problem.

## Can wild yam cream work on menopausal symptoms just as well as synthetic estrogen does?

Yes. But, wild yam cream commonly relieves the uncomfortable hot flashes, night sweats, insomnia, and mood swings without side effects or risks associated with synthetic estrogen drugs.

## How does natural progesterone differ from synthetic progesterone?

Synthetic progesterone is actually called progestogen and is a different chemical than progesterone. Since progestogen is a different molecule, it can't do what natural progesterone accomplishes.

## Will natural progesterone help ovarian cysts?

Yes, but be sure to see your doctor if you suspect you have cysts.

## Can I use natural progesterone without estrogen for preventing osteoporosis?

Yes. The effect of progesterone on bone and for treating osteoporosis has not been conclusively proven. Recent research indicates that progesterone is associated with an increase in bone formation, which may actually reverse the bone loss of osteoporosis.[14] However, studies in this area are conflicting and the controversy continues. Estrogen, commonly prescribed as a deterrent to osteoporosis, only slows down the process of bone loss. Some practitioners recommend a combination of estrogen and progestogen to prevent this condition. Others believe estrogen supplementation is not necessary at all for menopausal and postmenopausal women who still have their ovaries. Consult a health practitioner to determine your risk factors so you can make an informed decision about your treatment choices for osteoporosis.

## Can I use wild yam cream or natural progesterone cream if I have had a hysterectomy? Doesn't some form of estrogen need to be taken?

Before I answer this question, I want any woman considering a hysterectomy to seek a second opinion. This major surgery is one of the most popular operations performed in the United States—800,000 per year in 1984. Contrary to what you might think, this surgery is not without risks. Two thousand women die from hysterectomy complications each year. Others may suffer from fever, wound infections, hepatitis, urinary incontinence, bowel perforations or later on have adhesions (internal scars) causing intestinal obstructions, pain and other problems.[15]

If you've already had a complete hysterectomy (uterus and ovaries removed), most practitioners recommend starting with natural progesterone only and adding estrogen if no relief occurs within two weeks. If this isn't effective after three months, some low dose estrogen may be required, according to health practitioners.

If your hysterectomy involved the removal of your uterus only, then you have your ovaries and your body is still capable of producing estrogen and progesterone. Theoretically you shouldn't need supplemental hormones. However, according to Penny Wise Budoff, M.D., even a tubal ligation (female sterilization where a small piece of the fallopian tubes are cut out) can cause heavy menstrual bleeding or irregular periods. This is due to a change in ovarian function.[16] I'm sure the same thing could happen when a uterus-only hysterectomy is performed. Natural progesterone or wild yam cream may help in these situations. Ask your doctor.

## Should estrogen be used without natural progesterone?

Some practitioners believe natural progesterone is sufficient because in our society we produce or consume on overabundance of estrogen. It appears most women are estrogen dominant—their estrogen levels are higher than normal. In other words, the estrogen-progesterone teeter-totter is top heavy in favor of estrogen. Other practitioners believe it is extremely important to use natural progesterone along with any form of estrogen. This subject is very controversial. Without progesterone, estrogen may contribute to endometrial cancer. Estrogen taken alone may contribute to water retention, fibrocystic breast disease, fibroid tumors, and cysts in the ovarian area. Again, it really depends upon you and what is good for your body. See a health care practitioner to determine the choices best for your body.

# *I have gone through menopause and haven't taken any hormones. Do I need hormones?*

Probably not. Women who never had any menstrual problems are less likely to experience menopausal symptoms. Also, remember that hormonal replacement therapy is a relatively new treatment. So why is it that all of a sudden, every woman needs this remedy? If you're worried about health risks like heart disease and osteoporosis, work with a practitioner who can help you minimize your chances of developing these diseases using lifestyle maneuvers like diet and exercise. If you're plagued by menopausal symptoms, again look at your lifestyle. Also, remember the Japanese women who hardly suffer from hot flashes because of the soy foods they eat (and probably their healthier diet in general). If there is a history of osteoporosis in your family or if you have many of the risk factors like smoking and a sedentary lifestyle, consult your health professional.

# *I am taking hormones prescribed by my physician. Can I switch to a wild yam cream or natural progesterone cream? How do I do this?*

Yes. If you are using synthetic estrogen and/or progestogen, you can gradually switch by substituting wild yam cream or natural progesterone cream. Natural health practitioners say that after you begin applying the cream, it is recommended to gradually cut back each month on the synthetic supplements for three months. Half the dose the first month, half it again the second, and half of that dose the third month. However, since weaning off steroid hormones can have adverse affects, I urge you to do this with the knowledge and support of your doctor.

## I am post-menopausal. Will I begin menstruation again or experience breakthrough bleeding if I use natural progesterone cream?

Probably not with wild yam cream, and generally not with natural progesterone cream. It depends upon your age, your body and how much cream you use. If it does occur, you can cut back on your dosage. If bleeding persists for any length of time, discontinue the cream altogether and consult with your physician. You may be able to try the cream again with your doctor's help.

## Why does wild yam or natural progesterone cream help PMS?

PMS is often due to high levels of estrogen in the body which results in a low ratio of progesterone to estrogen. This ratio can be evened out by taking extra progesterone. Natural progesterone is very effective for many women suffering from hormonally based PMS. Most of the uncomfortable emotional, physical, and mental symptoms can be relieved. If your symptoms are especially severe, your doctor may recommend pharmaceutical doses of natural progesterone cream. Personally, and from the many women I've spoken with, wild yam cream is also very effective in treating PMS.

## Will wild yam cream or natural progesterone cream help amenorrhea (no periods)?

Yes. I've had many women tell me how their periods returned after using progesterone. However, like any condition, you need to know the cause before starting treatment. Amenorrhea can be caused by a number of things like anorexia nervosa, pituitary tumors and most commonly—pregnancy! If your periods have stopped and you don't know why, have a pregnancy test done before you use natural progesterone cream or any other treatment.

## *How do wild yam cream or natural progesterone cream help endometriosis and fibrocystic breast disease?*

These conditions have many contributing factors. However, if excess estrogen is circulating in the body, natural progesterone may help to balance out the estrogen to progesterone relationship.

## *What are the side effects of natural progesterone cream?*

Taken in the right amounts, natural progesterone cream is free from side effects. If you get overly enthusiastic and use more than the recommended amount of progesterone cream, then you might experience side effects like a change in your menstrual period. Women who use progesterone cream for irregular cycles may notice spotting during ovulation. With continued use, however, periods should become regular and spotting should cease. Post-menopausal women don't normally report any side effects. Natural progesterone may increase your thyroid activity. If you're taking thyroid medication or natural thyroid supplements, talk to your doctor. Again, if you have problems using progesterone, consult with a knowledgeable health care practitioner.

I hope I have answered all of your questions about the wild yam, a very wise yam! This question and answer journey was an education for me. One thing I learned was that natural medicine is about choices and options, in treatments good for you and your body. Once I realized this, I began to think about my own problems with PMS. The next step on my journey was finding out all I could about healing PMS with wild yam cream. I'll look into that dip in the road next, in Chapter Five.

# Summary

- Hormone-like compounds (called "phytohormones") are found in plants and foods.

- These "phytohormones" are thought to compete for receptor sites in your body with your naturally occurring hormones.

- Phytoestrogenic plants provide safe natural solutions for PMS, menopause and other female conditions.

- Natural progesterone, derived from wild yam, soybeans and wool fat, is identical to the progesterone occurring in your body.

- Wild yam contains diosgenin, a substance used to make natural progesterone and other steroid hormones in the laboratory.

- Natural progesterone is chemically different from progestogen.

- Wild yam doesn't contain actual hormones, but it is theorized that its diosgenin may have progesterone-like qualities and may even be used to make other hormones in your body. There is no evidence for this.

- According to women who have tried it, wild yam cream helps menstrual disorders, PMS and menopausal symptoms.

- Natural progesterone cream applied topically is the most

direct route into the bloodstream. Wild yam cream is thought to work the same way.

- FDA proposed amount of natural progesterone in a two ounce cosmetic cream jar is one milligram.

*Part Two*

# NEW DISCOVERIES FOR WOMEN'S HEALTH

# Chapter 5

# AM I GOING CRAZY? HEALING PMS

HAVE YOU EVER SUFFERED from Pre-Menstrual Syndrome (PMS)? Perhaps you have experienced these vague, hard-to-explain symptoms of PMS: bloating, headaches, food cravings, fatigue, irritability, depression, or backache. Your co-workers, husband or friends may think you're exaggerating about how debilitating these recurring monthly symptoms are. Any physically or emotionally stressful event can trigger PMS—consider marriage, divorce, pregnancy, promotion, moving, the death of a loved one, or such crises like an automobile accident. These events are part of life. Happy times or unpleasant experiences can stir-up your hormones and consequently, your life. Over 25 million women in the United States have suffered from PMS at some point in their lives. Certain experts report this number is much larger. You know the way you feel is real. You're not crazy. I questioned my own sanity until I found natural solutions that healed my wacky symptoms. Wild yam cream came to my rescue and saved me from the clutches of PMS.

I know first hand about stress-induced PMS, because I first experienced classic PMS symptoms after being involved in a car accident. Back then, of course, I never made the connection between the trauma of the accident to the onset of PMS. For years, I experienced depression, breast tenderness and bloating every two weeks before my period. I just assumed it was normal since so many women suffer from the same symptoms and so many more.

PMS is not a disease per se. It's a syndrome or waste basket of at least 150 emotional, physical and mental symptoms that appear every month around two weeks before your period. The frustration of this condition is you feel fine for a week or two after you menstruate, then the insanity of PMS hits you once again. This explains why you can feel on top of the world one week and in the very depths of hell the next. It took me eight years of living this way before I considered going to the doctor, and finally through this journey learned the link between my hormones, menstrual cycle and PMS.

# My Life With PMS

My monthly cycle ruled my life. If you've been struggling with PMS, then you can relate to my story. The first week of my cycle I felt great. I had energy morning, noon and night. I was in a great mood and I felt happy. The following week, my energy began sliding down hill and I tired easily. I started feeling irritable and slightly moody. About mid-cycle, my anxiety mounted and my breasts hurt. Frustration and temperamental outbursts turned me into the "Bride of Frankenstein."

The week before my period I became barely nice. I couldn't run from what was inside me—though I desperately wanted to. I was weepy, moody, bitchy, and puffy. My physical and emotional symptoms grew uncontrollably worse as my gloom grew into a deep painful depression. Even my skin broke out! Before PMS reared its ugly head, I never had a pimple, even as a teenager. I finally went to a dermatologist for my acne and he gave me skin medications. Of course, he didn't ask me about stress or any menstrual problems.

The day before my period was a killer. An intense total misery set in and I was ready to shoot myself or anyone else who crossed my path. I cried for no reason and snapped at everyone. The smallest difficulty set me off. Suicide seemed reasonable, though I never tried it. Instead, I stuffed myself and my hurt with chocolate or any other sweet things I could find. Unfortunately, this made me even more anxious because I didn't want to get fat. During this time, life was unbearable. Those moments seemed like forever. Wasn't I a joy to live with?

PMS wasn't my only problem. Twinges of pain cued the beginning of my period and hours of severe cramps. Finally, when the painful cramps stopped, I felt great. All the emotional and physical things I'd lived with totally disappeared. I was so happy for about a week— until it began all over again. My life was an emotional rollercoaster. Was this how life was supposed to be? It was time to feel good once again, time to seek help. My regular physician heard my list of complaints. He did a battery of tests to discover the cause of my complaints. All his tests came out normal. How could all my tests coming out "normal" when I felt awful?

During my check-up, my doctor suggested I use birth control pills to treat my problems. First, he believed it was the best way to prevent pregnancy. Second, he felt the multi-purpose actions of birth control pills would cure my ailments. He knew my family had a history of heart disease and cancer. Little did I know then the side effects of synthetic hormones would actually aggravate my PMS symptoms and increase my risk for this conditions. To me, this means I'm not a candidate for any estrogenic drugs.

He also prescribed anti-depressants for my "bummed out attitude" and the stresses of life. Though the anti-depressants dampened my anxiety and depression, they turned me into a walking zombie. I was not only very spacey, but still experiencing the water weight gain, cramps, and breast tenderness I'd gone to see my doctor for in the first place. Instead of uncovering the cause of my problems, my doctor

merely prescribed drugs to mask all my symptoms and ultimately create even more problems. Has something like this
happened to you?

# Enough Is Enough

I tried to ignore the combined side-effects of anti-
depressants and oral contraceptives. After three months of
feeling worse, I finally decided I'd had enough and stopped
taking all the pills. I knew I had to do something else. First, I
needed to answer the questions —What was wrong with me?
What could I do to feel better? Who can I turn to when the
doctors tell me there is nothing wrong? Fortunately, this all
happened at the same time the world of natural medicine
opened up to me. Repeatedly, natural health doctors advised
me to try wild yam cream. I was ready to take charge of my
health and research the effects of hormone imbalances and
the wild yam.

Once I finished my studies, I decided to try wild yam
cream to see if it really worked. With the help of several
herbalists and holistic doctors, I created my own formula of
wild yam cream with chaste tree berry, jojoba oil, apricot kernel, Vitamins A, D and E, and aloe vera—individualized for
the special needs of myself and my family.

My herbal formula was devised to heal and restore my
physical and mental well-being—to create beauty inside and
out. I wanted my new cream to help prevent illness and
strengthen me by balancing my body and bringing it into har-
mony with nature. I tried to include herbs that would realign
the upset estrogen and progesterone in my body, protect
against cancer, improve my pimply skin and remove lines and
wrinkles. I included antioxidant nutrients to guard against
chronic disease and the effects of aging, and vitamins to nourish my body. I experimented by using a variety of ingredients

in assorted concentrations for a gestation period of nine months. Finally a formula was born that worked for me.

My return to health was slow but powerful. It took a month before I noticed a difference in my symptoms. First my pimples went away. According to Dr. Raymond Peat, "Patients consistently report...that using progesterone at the first sign of a pimple stops the development at that stage, prevents the expected outbreak, and within a few days resulted in relatively clear skin."[1] A few cycles later, my emotional black cloud cleared away to sunny, peaceful skies. I lost weight and my physical symptoms went the way of my depression and moodiness. I finally felt really good again. Wild yam cream really worked for my PMS. I said good-bye to PMS! You can too!

# PMS Has A History (Or Is It Herstory)?

Although I have only known the meaning of PMS for three years, it has been studied as a physical illness since 1920. In 1931, PMS and its symptoms were first linked to excess estrogen. Researchers thought these high levels were caused by either diminished estrogen excretion and/or an overproduction of estrogen within the body.[2] Seven years later, low progesterone production and the estrogen-top-heavy balance between the two were added to the PMS equation.[3] In 1943, scientists found estrogen excretion was inhibited by a vitamin B deficiency.[4]

In 1974, a study demonstrated that three to six days before menstruation estrogen was higher and progesterone was lower in women with anxiety related symptoms.[5] Four years later, PMS-depression was tied to decreased estradiol and elevated progesterone during the second half of the menstrual cycle. Research in 1983 indicated estradiol counters the effect of progesterone.[6] The past decade has brought about incredible amounts of new research on PMS. Symptoms are now linked to different body systems, with hormones frequently as the cause.

Today, most authorities agree PMS is caused by imbalanced hormones. Some physicians believe there are other contributing factors including a diet high in animal fat, vitamin and mineral deficiencies, untreated low blood sugar, chronic yeast infections, stress, thyroid disease, adrenal gland dysfunction, and lower than normal levels of the hormone DHEA. After 65 years, we are still searching for answers.

# Making Sense Of PMS

The very nature of PMS makes it a very difficult condition to diagnose and manage. Noted researcher Guy Abraham, M.D., made your doctor's job a little easier by dividing PMS symptoms into four distinct groups. Each body of symptoms is easily identified by its nickname. For example PMS-A stands for all the PMS symptoms related to anxiety (A). PMS-C stands for craving symptoms. PMS-D indicates depression. PMS-H means hyper-hydration or water retention type symptoms like bloating and breast tenderness.[7]

**PMS-A (Anxiety Symptoms)** = Linked with high estrogen and low progesterone levels.
**Examples:** Anxiety, irritability, mood swings, nervous tension.

**PMS-C (Craving Symptoms)** = Linked to an increase in appetite and carbohydrate tolerance. Deficiency of prostaglandin PGE1 in some cases.
**Examples:** Increased appetite, headache, fatigue, dizziness or fainting, and heart palpitations.

**PMS-D (Depression)** = Linked to low estrogen, high progesterone, and elevated levels of androgens (if there is growth of facial hair).

**Examples:** Depression, crying, forgetfulness, confusion and insomnia.

**PMS-H (Hyper-Hydration)** = Linked with the hormone aldosterone.

**Examples:** Fluid retention, weight gain, swollen arms and legs, breast tenderness, and abdominal bloating.[8]

If you are suffering from any of these symptoms, PMS may be a part of your life.

## How Do You Know If You Officially Have PMS?

I attributed my behavior to PMS without having a professional diagnosis. If your symptoms fit into the definition below, you may have PMS. In her book, *Once a Month,* Hunter House, Dr. Katharina Dalton states, "It is essential to establish a definition of PMS for proper diagnosis. The definition of premenstrual syndrome is the presence of any symptoms or complaints that regularly come just before or during early menstruation, but are absent at other times of the cycle."[9] This precise definition means there are three requirements to be fulfilled for a correct diagnosis:

1. Symptoms must be present every month for at least three months.
2. Symptoms must be present premenstrually, and cannot start before ovulation.
3. There must be complete absence of symptoms after menstruation for a minimum of seven days.

A blood test can also help your doctor diagnose PMS. This test estimates the binding capacity of sex hormone binding globulin (SHBG).

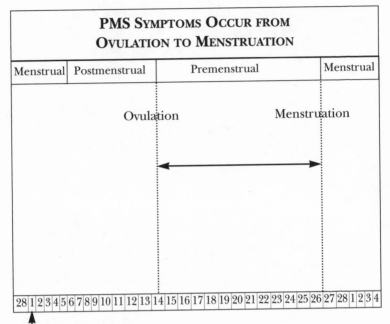

| Menstrual | Postmenstrual | Premenstrual | Menstrual |
|---|---|---|---|
| | | Ovulation           Menstruation | |

28 1 2 3 4 5 6 7 8 9 10 11 12 13 14 15 16 17 18 19 20 21 22 23 24 25 26 27 28 1 2 3 4

**↑**
**Day one of menstruation**

# Charting Your PMS Symptoms

If you want to discover if you have PMS on your own, you need to keep a chart of your symptoms. Writing down all your symptoms—physical, mental and emotional—will help you determine if you truly have PMS. It will also increase your understanding of how estrogen and progesterone (and other hormones) influence your symptoms.

Keeping a menstrual chart is easy to do. Record when your symptoms occur and to what degree, for at least two months. You begin by taking your basal body temperature every morning before you get out of bed. By recording your temperature, you will know when you ovulate and if your symptoms occur before or after ovulation. You can purchase a BBT thermometer along with instructions on how to use it from most drug stores. After you record your temperature, also write down any symptoms you may be experiencing. Notice if your symptoms follow a certain pattern during the month. Your temperature dips at mid cycle (at ovulation) and then rises. After that, your temperature should remain high until menstruation. If your temperature gradually decreases, your progesterone may be too low.[10]

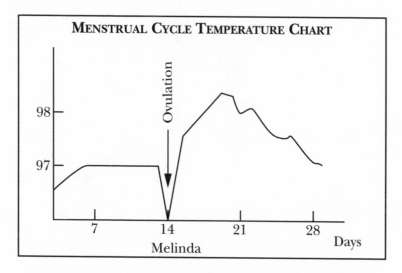

## What About Your Thyroid And PMS?

If you have PMS you may also have a thyroid or blood sugar problem. I think some low thyroid problems are hard to detect. Among the many tests my doctor did on me was a thyroid test. I had all the symptoms of low thyroid—feeling cold, puffy eyes, dry hair and skin. I even had to sleep with heavy socks to keep my feet warm. Yet my test results were still normal! Hypothyroid, or low thyroid, is one of the most widespread conditions for women. This condition remains undetected in over 40 percent of women. You may have a thyroid problem and not even know it. Hypothyroidism means the thyroid gland is producing smaller than normal amounts of thyroid hormone.

One study drew a correlation between abnormal thyroid function and PMS. It showed 94 percent of 54 PMS patients tested had thyroid dysfunction as compared with none of the 12 patients without PMS.[11] Hypothyroidism can have similar symptoms to PMS: fatigue, headaches, low sex drive, poor circulation and menstrual disturbances.

Dr. Broda Barnes of Littleton, Colorado speculates there is also a connection between hypothyroidism and low blood sugar. He says the liver is unable to release glycogen (the stored form of sugar) and produce glucose if your thyroid is underactive. This causes a low blood-sugar condition.

Dr. Barnes found a simple test to pinpoint hypothyroidism. Take your basal body temperature before getting out of bed each morning, as you do for detecting ovulation. A subnormal basal temperature of 97.8 degrees or lower indicates your thyroid may be sluggish. Repeat this test again during your period.

Dr. Peat says healthy thyroid function is essential for your body to use progesterone—either naturally occurring in your body or as a supplement. He sees a direct correlation between women who have breast cancer and the incidence of hypothyroidism and low progesterone. He believes the same women suffering from PMS will be most likely to suffer from menopausal symptoms, age related diabetes, and even breast cancer. I have personally seen the above hormone relationships, that Dr. Peat talks about, in action. One member of my family has breast cancer, thyroid problems as well as diabetes. How different her life would be today if a doctor, like Dr. Peat, had found the cause of her problems before they became major life threatening diseases.

A healthy thyroid needs many nutrients to function properly like vitamin A, selenium, zinc and iodine. Iodized salt is our most important source of iodine originally introduced to prevent cases of goiter, an enlargement of the thyroid often due to iodine deficiency. However, since then high iodine in salt and other foods has created almost the opposite problem.

Over the years, iodine consumption has increased dramatically through iodates (added to bakery products), FD&C Red Dye No. 3, some produce, contaminated dairy foods (from iodophor-disinfected pipes and containers, and iodine fed to cows as a foot rot prevention), fish and seaweed (we are eating more seafood), and nutritional supplements. When totaled up, Americans eat two to five times the RDA for iodine.

# Estrogen And Progesterone Levels Affect PMS

If estrogen and progesterone are at the bottom of your PMS, it's essential to balance out these hormones. However, other hormones are involved too, as are diet, lifestyle and stress. True healing of PMS demands that you and your doctor dig up the root cause of your problems. I want to concentrate on how estrogen and progesterone, the battling-balancing twins influence how you feel each month.

In Chapters Two and Three I talked about how your menstrual cycle works and the effects both estrogen and progesterone have on you and your period. Estrogen rules the first half of your cycle, while progesterone is the master of the second half—the two weeks just before your period when you usually feel horrible (if you have PMS). Estrogen in the right amounts makes you feel energetic, high amounts of progesterone can depress and tire you. It makes sense then that if estrogen rises too much, you'll feel anxious instead of exuberant —kind of like drinking too much coffee. If depression hits you premenstrually, then excessively high progesterone is probably dragging you down.

Have you ever over ate on foods like Twinkies™ or Ding Dongs™ before your period? It's not surprising, because higher progesterone levels increase cravings for carbohydrates, estrogen ups blood sugar levels and reduces your cravings. You really aren't crazy! There's a physiological explanation for your elusive symptoms. Your suffering is genuine, and so is the solution!

# Say Good Bye To PMS With Natural Progesterone!

Conventional treatments for PMS have included synthetic hormones like contraceptive pills, diuretics, counseling, tranquilizers and thyroid medications. Oral contraceptives and progestogen tend to worsen PMS symptoms because they lower your level of normal progesterone. There are very different side effects depending on the type of progestogen you use. There are no side effects with wild yam cream and rarely with natural progesterone made from the wild yam.[12]

How does natural progesterone help PMS? Over forty years ago a very smart doctor from England began to treat women with natural progesterone made from the wild yam. This doctor, Katharina Dalton, M.D., has been a true pioneer and authority on PMS research and treatment since 1953. She established the first PMS treatment center in London and has successfully treated over 30,000 women with natural progesterone in her clinic for over 30 years. In 1983, Dr. Dalton conducted a study using natural progesterone on 86 women with PMS. A remarkable 83 of her subjects reported complete relief of all of their symptoms.[13]

Dr. Dalton concluded progesterone receptors could be the "missing link" in understanding PMS. She states, "Either there are not enough progesterone receptors to transport the molecules of progesterone into the nucleus (of the cell), or the ability of the receptors is inhibited by adrenaline or some other unknown factor." Her comprehensive studies and treatment of thousands of women reveal that PMS is, in many cases, a progesterone related disease.

According to Susan Lark, M.D., "Synthetic progestins were used originally instead of natural progesterone because they can be taken orally. Unfortunately, natural progesterone cannot be ingested because it is destroyed during digestion and never reaches the bloodstream. In recent years, a new micronized form of progesterone is available that is protected from the stomach acid and enzymes and can be absorbed and used by the body. Made from the natural progesterone found in yams and soybeans, oral micronized progesterone has gained wide acceptance by physicians as a treatment for PMS. I began to prescribe natural progesterone a decade ago to my PMS patients and I am very pleased by the response to this treatment. It seems to be particularly helpful in controlling the emotional symptoms of PMS such as anxiety and mood swings."[14]

The best time to start using progesterone therapy is about two days before you expect PMS symptoms to begin (about day 14 to 16 days in a 28 day cycle), and continue therapy until menstruation. The exact amount and length of dosage will vary depending your cycle and symptoms. Do not use it during menstruation. If you choose to use natural progesterone, your physician can prescribe it for you either by injection, with a rectal or vagina suppository or as capsules.

# Mother Nature's Answers To PMS

If you have PMS, please know you don't have to live with it forever. My PMS responded well to easy-to-use wild yam cream. It not only worked for my PMS symptoms, but it helped smooth out my wrinkles and made me look younger.

Karen Lee Torell, D.C. from Newport Beach, California, has used wild yam cream both personally and for her patients.

She writes: "My personal experience...has shown it to entirely eliminate all premenstrual symptoms, forcing me to observe the calendar more closely to remember when to stop using the creme (sic) to allow for my period. However, the creme does not stop my normal cycle from occurring should I forget to discontinue it at the 26-27 day (my normal cycle). I have used the creme (sic) for over 18 months, without any negative results! I am 47 years old, my hormone levels are excellent, with no indication of approaching menopause." Dr. Torell also reports her patients benefit from using wild yam cream for excessive menstrual bleeding, tender breasts, irregular periods, hot flashes, birth control pill withdrawal, and mild to moderate cases of endometriosis.

Since discovering this great plant, my mind has opened up to other forms of natural healing. In addition to using wild yam cream, I changed my diet, exercised more, and took vitamins with minerals. It is up to you to find the right combination of therapies that will heal your PMS.

## Amie's PMS story

Amie had suffered from PMS symptoms for many years. Bloating irritability and anxiety were her biggest complaints. She began using wild yam creme twice a day from ovulation to the day before her period. After she had been using the wild yam creme for one and one half months she noticed her PMS bloating and irritability disappeared.

## Diet

Did you know something as simple as changing your diet can drastically improve your PMS symptoms? I found a diet high in complex carbohydrates (vegetables, whole grains, legumes) gave me energy, leveled out my blood sugar and wiped out my PMS. Unlike sugary treats, foods rich in fiber and complex carbohydrates prevent your blood sugar from bouncing up and down like a beach ball. Eating six small well-balanced meals each day, about three hours apart, also helps maintain the blood sugar levels.

I know this sounds difficult to some of you, but try it and see how you feel. Enduring low blood sugar is even worse with the irritability, fatigue, and shaking that comes with it. A study published in 1982 found PMS patients consumed more refined carbohydrates like white sugar and white flour, and dairy products than the PMS-free control group. The control group ate a diet higher in B vitamins, iron, zinc, and manganese. These findings demonstrated the importance of diet in PMS treatment.[15] However, it goes the other way too. Unbalanced hormones tend to egg on food cravings. Hormones can "stir-up" both you and your diet!

## Exercise

Exercise is beneficial for your health and your hormones. If you exercise aerobically at least 20 to 30 minutes, three times a week, you can reduce stress and improve your blood flow. Adrenaline, the fight-or-flight hormone released during tense times, can trigger headaches and irritability when stress levels soar. Something as simple as walking around the block on a regular basis can improve your sense of well being—at any age.

## Vitamin and mineral supplements

Certain vitamins and minerals can reduce your PMS symptoms. Look at the chart in Appendix B for more information. Many physicians recommend supplements of vitamin B-6 and B complex, calcium and magnesium and a multi-vitamin. Vitamin B-6 reduces water retention, calms nervous tension, and preserves your magnesium levels. Magnesium normalizes glucose metabolism, and calms your nerves. Calcium reduces pelvic pain, insomnia, bloating, and nervousness. Vitamin E reduces breast pain and tenderness, and normalizes production of sex hormones. Vitamin C reduces allergic response, and relieves pain. Lecithin helps prevent excessive fatty deposits in the liver, and deactivates estrogen. Zinc improves glucose tolerance and helps regulate prostaglandins. I have tried all of them. I notice a huge improvement in the way I feel emotionally and physically especially when I take magnesium.

# Natural Solutions For PMS Symptoms

You have many natural treatment selections for your PMS symptoms. To make coping with these choices a little less stressful, I've compiled a list of common PMS symptoms as well as suggested natural remedies. Also, browse through Appendix C: Hormonal Materia Medica to learn more about each remedy. Say good-bye to PMS forever!

## *Headaches, anxiety and mood swings*

These symptoms usually occur when estrogen levels are high and progesterone is low. The herbs suggested help release stress and muscle tension, and balance your hormones.

**Natural Solutions:** Wild yam cream, natural progesterone, licorice, dong quai, ginseng, kava, chaste tree berry, passion flower.

## *Fatigue and lack of energy*

These symptoms can be caused by exhausted adrenal glands. Herbal combinations that encourage and support the adrenal glands without stimulants can be beneficial.

**Natural Solutions:** Sarsaparilla, licorice root, natural progesterone, wild yam cream, uva ursi, rose hips, ginger, capsicum, panothenic acid (B-5).

## *Water retention and breast tenderness*

Aldosterone, the hormone that controls water and salt metabolism, is involved with these symptoms.

**Natural Solutions:** Wild yam cream, natural progesterone, dandelion, kelp, licorice.

## *Hypoglycemia*

This is low blood sugar. Highly refined carbohydrate foods aggravate this condition by causing a surge of insulin into the blood stream and a resulting plummet in blood sugar.

**Natural Solutions:** Wild yam cream, natural progesterone. If you are hypothyroid, these thyroid supporting herbs may help (check with your doctor first). Kelp, kombu, dulse, alfalfa, Irish moss, watercress, spirulina, borage, nettles.

## *Donna's story*

> Donna discovered through a holistic medical practice and chiropractic care that she suffered from upset progesterone levels in her body. She was having trouble with very dry irritated skin, depression, hair loss with crushing fatigue and muscle soreness. She began using a wild yam cream recommended by her chiropractor. Since using it, all her symptoms have decreased and her dry skin has noticeably improved. Donna's skin glows and it is soft now.

**Natural Solutions:** Wild yam cream, natural progesterone, dandelion, kelp, licorice.

## Fibrocystic breast disease

Fibrocystic breast disease is a common breast condition occurring in 20 to 40 percent of women. This premenstrual breast pain and tenderness occurs in both breasts every cycle a week or two before a woman's period. For this reason, FBD is considered part of PMS.

A high estrogen to progesterone ratio is accepted as the cause, sometimes combined with an underactive thyroid. Many women develop FBD from ages 30 to 39, ten years before menopause when the progesterone levels begin to decrease. Fibroids usually disappear after menopause. Women with fibrocystic breasts are three times more likely to develop breast cancer.

Caffeine, found in black tea, coffee, some soft drinks and chocolate, appears to be a principal contributing factor. Thomas J. Finneran, D.C., a chiropractor from Newhall, California, recommends a daily massage to relieve breast fibroids. He suggests massaging each breast in a circular pattern with wild yam cream, olive oil or natural progesterone cream. Rub the right breast counter clockwise, and the left breast clockwise for maximum benefit.

**Natural solutions:** Wild yam cream, natural progesterone cream, chaste tree berry, licorice, dong quai, dandelion, burdock, yellow dock, alfalfa.

# Other Problems, Other Solutions

## Menstrual pain and cramps

This condition, called dysmenorrhea, affects up to half of all menstruating women. Although menstrual cramps are sometimes lumped in with PMS, dysmenorrhea is an entirely different condition. This is a complex and not entirely understood condition. Prostaglandins, hormones, anatomy, diet, exercise and stress all seem to play a part.

**Natural Solutions:** Wild yam cream, natural progesterone cream, chaste tree berry, valerian, passion flower, raspberry leaf, licorice root, motherwort, black haw.

## *Uterine bleeding disorders*

This circumstance includes excessive bleeding and spotting; delayed or suppressed menstruation. High levels of estrogen or low progesterone can aggravate these conditions. Bleeding can also be a sign of more serious problems like uterine fibroids or polyps, or cancer of the cervix or womb. If heavy bleeding lasts for more a month, check with your physician. Many doctors prescribe progestogens for heavy bleeding associated with low progesterone levels. Low fat diet and non-dairy diets are helpful, too.

**Natural Solutions:** Wild yam cream, natural progesterone cream, chaste tree berry, yellow dock, sarsaparilla, peony.

## *Endometriosis*

Endometriosis means endometrial tissue (the lining of the uterus) that grows in areas other than the uterus. There is no known cause for this very painful, crampy and abnormal bleeding condition. As this condition develops, the pain becomes progressively worse and begins earlier in the menstrual cycle. Dr. John Lee prescribes natural progesterone to his patients with mild to moderate endometriosis. Natural progesterone is used from day 10 to day 26 monthly and the dosage is increased until pelvic pains decreases. The treatment is continued for three to five years. None of Dr. Lee's patients with mild to moderate endometriosis have had to resort to surgery.[16]

**Natural Solutions:** Lady's mantle, hops, wild yam cream, natural progesterone cream, black haw, licorice, black cohosh, chaste tree berry, ginger, angelica root, chamomile, squaw vine.

## *Ovarian cysts*

Ovarian cysts are small fluid-filled, non-cancerous lumps on the ovary. The symptoms include abdominal pressure, pain, discomfort and bleeding with ovulation. Women who don't get their period or are bleeding excessively may have ovarian cysts. Usually, the cause is estrogen dominance.

**Natural Solutions:** Wild yam cream, natural progesterone cream, chaste tree berry, dandelion, burdock, white bryony.

## *Infertility*

Infertility may be due to low progesterone levels or high estrogen. Check with your doctor for the cause of your infertility.

**Natural Solutions:** Wild yam cream, natural progesterone, chaste tree berry, sarsaparilla, vervain, Siberian ginseng, lady's mantle, black haw, dandelion, cramp bark, spearmint, sarsaparilla, black cohosh, false unicorn root, licorice root, motherwort, dong quai.

## Summary

- PMS is treatable!

- There are over 150 recognized and documented symptoms.

- One cause of PMS is low levels of progesterone or high estrogen.

- PMS can also be the result of high progesterone and low estrogen.

- PMS can be categorized into four groups: PMS-A (anxiety), PMS-C (cravings), PMS-D (depression) and PMS-H (water retention).

- True PMS occurs after ovulation on a monthly basis.

- Low thyroid may be related to PMS.

- Develop a good exercise program and healthy diet to treat PMS.

- Natural solutions include wild yam cream, natural progesterone cream, herbs and vitamins.

# Chapter 6

# WHAT IS MENOPAUSE ANYWAY?

IF YOU ARE ONE of the baby boom generation who is turning middle aged in the year 2000, you are part of the 55 million women who are moving from a monthly menstrual cycle to the process we call menopause. Imagine over 55 million women with raging hormones stirring up the world! That kind of activity could cause a major revolution!

I have come to realize that this stage of my life is just around the corner. Just like you know as a teenager you're going to get your period someday, menopause is part of our female life experience. What happens in menopause? What can you except? Hot flashes! Night sweats and more! In Chapter Four, I explained how wild yam cream helps women with their menopausal symptoms. In fact I believe 90 percent of women I talk to who use wild yam cream do so to relieve their hot flashes. If you have hot flashes, you know you would do just about anything to be more comfortable. From my experience, not all wild yam creams work. That's why I sent my cream formula to be tested on women to ensure it works. As a result of all my testing, one woman wanted to call it the Miracle Cream!

## Is Menopause A Stop On The Highway, an Exit Ramp Or Transition Lane?

The way I look at menopause and most other women do,

is that it's a transition lane in life. Your monthly periods stop and your ability to bear children exits, but your life definitely goes on, despite hormonal changes. During this transition lane, many women experience discomfort as certain hormonal levels decline—causing physical, emotional and mental symptoms. Over 85 percent of menopausal women in the United States suffer from at least some uncomfortable symptoms.

Menopause is clinically defined as the permanent, natural cessation of menstruation. Today, hysterectomies produce artificially induced menopause. Either way, you know you are menopausal when menstruation has stopped for at least six months. Menopause affects approximately 3,500 women each day! Each year over 1 million women in the United States naturally experience menopause. The hormone revolution is starting!

For years, we have been blitzed by news reports and told by health professionals—"You don't have to suffer from menopausal symptoms like hot flashes, insomnia and night sweats." For the most part, the only choice offered has been estrogen replacement therapy (ERT). "Pop a pill to make all your cares go away." I call this estrogen mania. Since the 1970s, frightening reports of the cancer hazards from ERT have prompted many women to question whether the risks are worth the benefits. During my journey of discovery, I learned many women are concerned about how to manage their hormones during menopause and remain disease-free without the risks and side-effects of ERT. Fortunately, I found wild yam cream and other natural solutions can restore equilibrium without ERT's jeopardy.

## Are You Ready For A Hot Flash?

Menopause really hit close to home for me one day. My 55 year old mother and I were having lunch. Suddenly, I witnessed a wave of pink creep across her neck and face. Then, her color changed to beet red. *Something is wrong with her,* I thought. Beads of perspiration drenched her forehead. The red flush spread from her face and neck up to her hairline. She said, "Feel me. I am all wet and sweaty. My clothes are all wet. I am having palpitations!" As she wiped the heavy sweat from her face, she complained, "The hair on my head is soaking wet. Is it hot in here?" I replied, "Mom, it's 50 degrees below zero outside! Hot it isn't, unless you go south to Florida. It's freezing outside and it's cold inside this room. This is the wrong season to be hot." Then Mom said, "I've got the chills. It feels cold in here now." I couldn't believe what I was hearing. I jumped up and shouted, "Are you okay? Are you sick?" She replied "No, I am not sick. It's just a hot flash. It will pass." All I could think to say was, "Does this mean you have hot news?"

## The Transition Lane

Although menopause doesn't set in until you're between ages 46 to 53, estrogen begins to decline over a 10 to 15 year span beginning any time from your late 40's through 50's. This is your body's preparation for the day when estrogen levels are so low that menstruation finally stops. Once your period disappears, estrogen continues to drop as you age into your 70's and 80's. Medically, a woman is considered menopausal when she has no period for 6 to 12 months after age 45.

## The Four Phases Of Menopause

Menopause is divided into four phases beginning around 40 years old. The whole process, from your 40's to your 70's, is called climacteric.

1. Premenopause begins around age 40.
2. Perimenopause lasts for two to four years when female sex hormones are changing.

3. Menopause is when menstruation actually ceases.
4. Postmenopause is when your body has adjusted to new hormonal levels.

Changes occur with the four main hormones that orchestrate the menstrual cycle— estrogen, progesterone, follicle stimulating hormone (FSH) and luteinizing hormone (LH). Your ovaries and adrenal glands produce estrogen and progesterone during your fertile years. The adrenal glands make estrogen by converting the male hormone, androstenedione, to estrogen—especially before puberty and once again in mid-life when the ovaries no longer produce sufficient amounts. Fat cells also manufacture estrogen—so if you have more fat cells, you make more estrogen. Research indicates thinner women tend to experience earlier menopause.

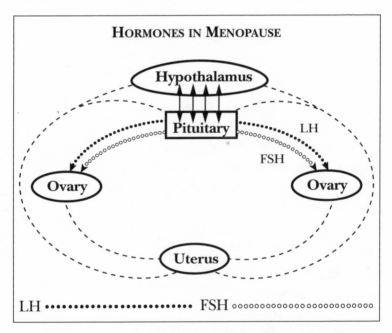

Women are born with a limited amount of follicles that eventually become eggs. Each month for 30 to 40 years, women menstruate and the eggs either die or become fertilized. After age 40, fewer follicles mature each month, and the ones that do are less sensitive to hormones. As a result, cycles shorten or become irregular.

By the time a woman reaches her late 40's or early 50's, the follicles have degenerated to the point where they produce so little estrogen that conception becomes difficult or impossible. At the same time FSH levels increase in an attempt to bolster diminishing estrogen. (Kind of like kicking a car that doesn't start. It feels good, but doesn't help much.) Toward the end of the menopausal change, the follicles' ability to produce eggs is exhausted, and estrogen level drops until there is not even enough to build up the lining of the uterus to start menstruation and menopause begins.

# How Does The Transition Affect You?

After age 40, you may begin to notice subtle changes caused by hormonal alterations, such as drier skin, new wrinkles, frequent urination, depression and moodiness. At first you may become aware that your periods are irregular and monthly blood flow is thinner or thicker. You may notice changes in your cervical mucus during ovulation. Eventually some of the more obvious symptoms may appear: hot flashes, night sweats, vaginal dryness, mood swings, headaches, irritability, insomnia, weight changes and fatigue. Some of these symptoms you may already have experienced as PMS—all are due to hormonal changes.

There are several health problems associated with the decline of estrogen in menopause, such as increased risk of osteoporosis, cancer, heart attacks, changes in blood vessel walls and stroke. The top two causes of death for post-menopausal women are heart disease and cancer. Medical professionals are beginning to realize, however, that some of these problems can be successfully handled with diet, exercise and healthy living.

Some women sail through menopause and others suffer symptoms for years. The symptoms and intensity vary greatly with each woman. Are you shocked? I mean really, why should your menopause be exactly the same as your best friend's? Was your menstrual period? I remember that I just hated to know my best friend got her period in seventh grade and mine didn't arrive until practically the end of eighth. Of course, maybe her menopause will be first, too!

# Symptoms Of The Menopause Transition

"Will I get menopausal symptoms?"—is a question many women ask themselves. I know I do. Researchers reveal there are certain characteristics associated with who is more or less likely to suffer from menopausal symptoms. You are less likely to suffer symptoms during menopause if you are well-educated, began menstruating late, have never married or had children and are in a high income bracket. Women more likely to experience symptoms have suffered from PMS, and have had a hysterectomy (artificial menopause).[1] Here's a comprehensive list of possible menopausal symptoms. Remember, you probably won't get all of these.

**Physical**

Hot flashes.
Night sweats.
Heart palpitations.
Itching skin.
Irregular or heavy menstrual periods.
Menstrual periods stop.
Vaginal dryness or itching.
Backaches.
Bone loss.
Muscular weakness.

Sagging breasts.
Dry skin and wrinkles.
Hair loss or thinning.
Facial hair.
Migraine headaches.
Varicose veins.

**Emotional**

Depression.
Mood swings.
Insomnia.
Decreased sex drive.
Nervousness.
Forgetfulness (I almost didn't remember this one!)

# Wild Yam Cream And Replacement Therapies

To use hormonal replacement therapy or not is one of the most important decisions we as women face in our lives. Natural solutions can and should be your first choice. Remember, start simple, if that doesn't work, then work your way up to more complex therapies.

The risk of disease versus the benefits of ERT, or synthetic estrogen taken alone, weighs heavily in the minds of many women. Hormonal replacement therapy refers to a combination therapy of synthetic estrogen and progestogen, those famous two balancing hormones we all must respect. If you are aware of the risks of HRT and ERT, both short and long-term, you can make a decision that is right for you. Replacement therapy is really a misnomer, because it does not actually replace your own natural hormones—your hormones are supposed to decline at this time of your life—but rather, it adds extra hormones that don't necessarily act the same way as your own estrogen and progesterone do.

In Chapters Three and Four, I explained replacement therapies and the wild yam. Here I want to review the benefits of wild yam cream and natural progesterone. First, remember wild yam in cream form is used as a whole herb. You receive multiple benefits from using the whole herb. Second, since decreasing and sometimes flucutating hormones is the reason for menopausal symptoms, it makes sense that balancing them will ease your transition.

Most doctors prescribe synthetic estrogen and/or progestogen for relief of menopausal symptoms. I've found wild yam, available in liquid, capsules or cream, to be a viable alternative. My favorite form is the cream. If you have never used a medicinal herbal cream before, then you will be pleasantly surprised with its effectiveness. Natural progesterone creams work on the same principle as estrogen patches—that is through skin receptors cells and absorbing directly into your bloodstream without going through your digestive system. (Hormones are broken down too quickly by digestion to make them optimally useful as oral medicines.) I use wild yam in cream form, based on the above principles.

I've found it takes anywhere from one day to four months to see results with wild yam cream. It depends on your system. Usually, you'll notice a difference in a few days. Menopausal women apply wild yam cream for two to three weeks and stop during menstruation (if they're still having periods). If you are still experiencing some problems, you can try wild yam cream containing natural progesterone. If this treatment doesn't work for you, try a cream with licorice root or other helpful medicinal herbs as well. If that still doesn't help, ask your physician about prescribing stronger doses of natural progesterone for you. Finally, if all these natural therapies fail, then consider synthetic hormones. Also, remember the importance of professional medical guidance throughout this time. It's very difficult to diagnose yourself and to know what therapies are best. If one doctor isn't helping you, you may also want to search for another. Treatments vary in effectiveness, as do physicians.

## *ERT And HRT*

There are benefits to ERT and HRT, but there are also risks you need to know. It is estimated that over 80 percent of women seek natural alternatives for hormone replacement therapy because they will not or can not take estrogen replacement therapy. You are at risk years after you discontinue estrogen therapy. A recent study followed 5,563 postmenopausal women for nine years—one group took estrogen alone (ERT), and the other group was on estrogen and progesterone (HRT). The women taking estrogen alone had a six times higher incidence of endometrial cancer up to five years versus those using HRT. This risk is 15 times greater among long-term users. Women taking estrogen had the highest rate of cancer, followed by women taking no supplementation, with women taking progesterone having the lowest incidence of cancer.

Estrogen does relieve many of the common menopausal symptoms like hot flashes and vaginal dryness, and may protect you against heart disease and osteoporosis. However, it could cost you in the long run. Dr. Susan Lark states, "Estrogen is not a cure...because the hot flashes may return when replacement therapy is discontinued—the ovaries are not revitalized or regenerated in any way by ERT."[2]

Some of the common side-effects of estrogen replacement therapy are vaginal bleeding and spotting, menstrual cramps, PMS-like symptoms, no period, vaginal yeast infection, breast tenderness, nausea, vomiting, abdominal cramps and bloating, jaundice, hair loss, facial hair, skin rash, intolerance to contact lenses, headaches including migraines, dizziness, depression, increase or decrease in weight and changes in libido.

ERT may also increase your risk of endometrial and breast cancers, liver and gallbladder disease, elevated blood pressure (which can cause heart attacks or stroke) and blood clotting, especially if you are overweight. In higher doses, ERT can increase your risk of diabetes because it changes glucose levels. If you are already diabetic and taking estrogen, you should have your blood sugar levels monitored carefully.

HRT consists of both estrogen and progesterone. This combination was developed in recent years to help prevent osteoporosis, protect against heart disease and relieve the menopausal symptoms. The side-effects from progestogens sound an awful lot like PMS—water retention, nausea, anxiety, tender breasts, weight gain, vaginal discharge, irregular bleeding, bloating and headaches.

Some British researchers suggest that HRT is addictive, claiming PMS, postpartum depression and menopausal depression are evidence that female hormones alter mood. HRT can promote feelings of well-being and some women on HRT show signs of drug dependency. In light of this, blanket HRT prescriptions for all menopausal women over long periods of time could be dangerous.[3]

# Hysterectomy-induced Menopause

A full hysterectomy—removal of your ovaries and usually uterus—produces artificial menopause. There are thousands of hysterectomies performed in the United States every year. After a hysterectomy, a woman goes through emotional, physical and hormonal shock. She can be overcome with emotional problems and symptoms just like PMS—the feelings of depression, a sense of loss, a feeling of unworthiness and even headaches. She may not prepare for the emotional feelings of loss from the removal of her ovaries and uterus, often feeling she is no longer a whole woman. She also can suffer from menopausal symptoms.

The physical changes women experience after a hysterectomy are:

> For the first six to eight days after surgery there is an increase in follicle stimulating hormone (FSH) from the pituitary gland—just like during natural menopause.

> For the next eight to ten days there is an increase in the luteinizing hormone (LH).

> For 10 to 31 days, the FSH continues to increase to three times its previous amount and the LH doubles, remaining high for many years.

> For six to twelve months after surgery, the normal cyclical symptoms of PMS prior to the hysterectomy return.

I know about hysterectomy-induced menopause because I had the unhappy privilege of watching my sister suffer through it. During my journey of research I learned about the side-effects of ERT and how they were affecting my sister. While questioning natural medical practitioners, I asked them for a natural solution for her. She had her hysterectomy when she was only 30 years old and for over ten years dealt with the side-effects of ERT. Read about Leslie's story in Chapter 8.

# Welcome To Natural Solutions During Menopause

Let's begin with preventive measures to reduce your chance of menopausal symptoms even starting. Then, we will discuss natural solutions for some specific occurrences associated with the life transition we call menopause.

Fortunately, there are many safe solutions available for menopausal women including wild yam cream and other herbs, natural progesterone cream, diet, exercise and stress reduction. You can boost your natural hormone pool some-what using herbs, supplements and lifestyle habits. The risk of osteoporosis, cancer and heart disease can be significantly decreased through a natural approach with dietary and lifestyle changes. You don't need to raise your risk of breast and endometrial cancers in order to prevent these diseases.

## *Diet And Nutrition*

Preventing menopausal symptoms begins with a close exami-nation of your diet. Good nutrition leads to good health. Dr. John Lee sums it up: "We have now come to the crux of the problem. Healthy, well nourished follicle cells produce a healthy balance of estrogen and progesterone. Follicle cell dysfunction from any cause, especially from intracellular nutri-tional deficiencies and/or toxins, will lead to progesterone deficiency and estrogen dominance combined with elevated FSH and LH levels and hypothalamic hyperactivity."[4]

Eating well can go a long way, especially if good nutri-tion is practiced in early years. You can feel better during menopause by making some adjustments to your diet now. Eating a diet low in fat and animal protein, with plenty of fresh vegetables and fruit, whole grains and legumes can help eliminate some of the symptoms of menopause, as well as reduce your risk of cancer and heart disease.

Choose your diet wisely. Foods to avoid are sugar, fried and fatty foods, salty foods, dairy products (especially when high in fat), white flours, refined and processed foods, caf-feine, carbonated soft drinks, red meat and alcohol. If you're suffering from hot flashes, avoid hot and spicy foods. This makes perfect sense if you stop to think twice about it. Why drink hot coffee or eat spicy Mexican food if your body feels as if someone just put you in a sauna? Foods to include in your diet—black beans, sesame seeds, soybeans and other soy products, walnuts and peanuts, mulberries, yams, apples, cherries, olives, plum, carrots, whole grains (brown rice, barley, oats, wheat), carrots, celery, parsley and beets.

## *Nutritional Supplements Can Ease Your Transition*

Nutritional supplements are beneficial to ease the transition and symptoms of menopause. Naturopathic doctors recommended you supplement with Vitamin E, Vitamin B complex, B-6, Vitamin C and bioflavonoids, magnesium, boron, evening primrose oil and borage oil.

At the USDA's research facility in Grand Forks, North Dakota, Forrest Nielsen, Ph.D., has done some ground breaking studies on the effects of a relatively obscure mineral, boron. In postmenopausal women fed three milligrams of boron each day, estrogen rose equivalent to "levels found in women on estrogen replacement therapy."[5] Boron supplementation also decreased calcium lost through their urine by 40 percent.[6] Dark green, leafy vegetables, fruits (not citrus), nuts and legumes all contain boron. If you decide to take boron supplements, consult with a physician. Too much boron could increase your risk of osteoporosis.[7]

Vitamin E relieves hot flashes. One study noted 800 IU a day of Vitamin E relieved some women's hot flashes within two days. When the Vitamin E was combined with two to three grams per day of Vitamin C and one gram per day of calcium (administered in divided doses throughout the day), many women reported their hot flashes disappeared immediately. After one week, the Vitamin E was reduced to a maintenance level of 400 IU a day. Vitamin E in combination with B-6 was also found to ease breast pain. B-complex, 25-50 milligrams per day, was found to lessen moodiness.[8]

If you decide to try these vitamins, my only warning is to be careful with Vitamin B-6. Don't take more than 100 mg per day unless under the care of a nutrition-wise physician. Too much Vitamin B-6 can cause numbness and tingling in your hands and feet, a sign of peripheral neuropathy. If you experience these symptoms while on Vitamin B-6, discontinue taking it right away.

## Phytoestrogenic Herbs

Phytoestrogens are plant and herbs that contain estrogen-like substances. There are no long-term, well-controlled studies on the effects of phytoestrogens and other natural hormone sources. Most of the evidence we have at this point is based on clinical observations. Therefore, naturopathic physicians and other natural health practitioners disagree about when and how long phytoestrogens should be used.

These botanicals do not appear to cause side-effects. However, many physicians follow certain guidelines when prescribing them. If a woman is pregnant, has abnormal vaginal bleeding, thrombophlebitis or a history of this, phytoestrogens should be avoided. If she has a history of a related disorder connected with estrogen use, cancer related to estrogen use, or known or suspected breast cancer, any type of estrogen—including a natural source—should not be used.[9]

## Coffee And Cigarettes

There is also evidence that lifestyle can influence a woman's natural estrogen levels. One study discovered smoking altered the breakdown of estrogen in the liver and subsequently lowered one form of estrogen in the blood.[10] Another investigation revealed a relationship between increased caffeine intake and decreased free estrogen.[11]

# Natural Relief For The Main Menopausal Symptoms

## *Hot Flashes*

Over 80 percent of our American sisters experience hot flashes during the menopause transition. A hot flash means you have a sudden wave of extreme warmth and heat occurring any time, any place without warning causing heavy sweating. Hot flashes can last 30 seconds or longer. The frequency of hot flashes varies between daily, hourly, monthly or yearly, depending on, you guessed it, YOU.

The exact cause of hot flashes is uncertain. Several factors contribute to hot flashes—the ratio between estrogen and progesterone, being thin or not, a high fat diet, stress, weather, alcohol, caffeinated foods like coffee and chocolate, spicy foods and emotions. Foods high in phytoestrogens may also reduce your hot flashes.

There are many theories and studies about the causes of hot flash, sometimes called flushes. According to Penny Wise Budoff, M.D., in her book *No More Hot Flashes,* "Each hot flush is related directly to a pulsatile surge in LH production by the pituitary." A direct cause of hot flashes is hypothalamic factors regulating the releasing LH. The LH itself does not cause hot flashes. "This ties in hot flushes with hormonal disturbances in the hypothalamus, the heat-regulatory center of the brain."[12]

Susan Lark, M.D., suggests another hypothesis. She says that hot flashes occur when the estrogen receptors in the hypothalamus do not receive enough stimulation. In response, they may release a chemical substance that produces the hot flashes and other blood vessel reactions. The hypothalamus normally controls the body's temperature.[13]

Dr. John Lee believes, "Hot flushes are not a sign of estrogen deficiency, per se, but are due to heightened hypothalamic activity (vasomotor ability), secondary to low levels of estrogen and progesterone which, if raised, would produce a negative feedback effect to the pituitary and hypothalamus. Once progesterone levels are raised, estrogen receptors in these areas become more sensitive and hot flushes usually subside. The validity of this mechanism can be tested by measuring FSH and LH levels before and after adequate progesterone supplementation."[14]

Finnish researchers noted that Japanese who ate a traditional diet low in fat and high in soy foods such as tofu and miso excreted as much as 1000 more phytoestrogens in their urine as American women. This means that Japanese women consume considerably more phytoestrogens in their diet—one reason why hot flashes and other menopausal symptoms may be less frequent in that country.[15]

Lafayette Clinic and Wayne State University School of Medicine in Detroit used a breathing technique to relieve hot flashes consisting of slow deep breaths. This method reduced 33 women's hot flashes by 50 percent over a 24 hour period. The theory behind this therapy is breathing lowers the arousal of the central nervous system that normally occurs at the beginning of a hot flash. You can do this simple technique at home—take six to eight deep breaths per minute all the way down to your chest or abdomen. To prevent hot flashes from occurring in the first place, practice breathing this way twice a day for 15 minutes each time.[16]

If hot flashes drench you, dress in layers using natural fibers that breath. This way you won't get as hot and can remove clothing as the flash heats you up. Avoiding caffeine and alcohol can decrease the severity of hot flushes. Drinking plenty of water may help, too.

## Nancy's Story: Instant hot flash!

Nancy was working at a convention trade show. She

was under stress, drinking coffee and she began having hot flashes, night sweats, and insomnia. She could barely work the show. She was desperate to find relief instantly. She found the wild yam cream and began using the it twice a day a 1/2 teaspoon morning and night. Within two to three days, her night sweats, insomnia and hot flashes were disappeared. She discovered instant relief and was able to return to working comfortably.

Other natural solutions include wild yam cream, natural progesterone cream, chaste tree berry, motherwort, devils clubs, licorice root, black cohosh, blue cohosh, ginseng, dong quai, sarsaparilla, false unicorn root, fenugreek, dandelion, squaw vine, damiana, garden sage, violet, elder flower, milk thistle, bioflavonoids, cranberry extract, cherries, rose hips, bilberries, apple pectin and fennel.

## *Vaginal Dryness*

Did you know as you go through menopause, your vaginal walls may be thinning as your hormonal levels decrease? The result is atrophic vaginitis, vaginal dryness and itching, a major complaint among menopausal women.

Without wild yam cream or another effective treatment, vaginal dryness can cause irritation during sexual activity because a dry vagina tends to create painful friction during intercourse. This problem can be compounded by a hormonally induced decline in libido. However, when older married women are compared to older married men, the percentage who has sex is almost identical.

The pH levels in the vagina may also change, increasing your risk of infections. There are, however, some safe remedies for this problem. Lubricants provide moisture such as Replens (or K-Y Jelly), as well as Vitamin E oil or suppositories. Dr. John Lee recommends using natural progesterone cream to correct vaginal dryness. If this doesn't work, he suggests using intravaginal estriol cream available as a prescription from your doctor.

Many herbs and nutrients can help improve vaginal moisture and lubrication by increasing blood flow to uterine tissue. Essential fatty acids taken as evening primrose oil or borage oil might help. Other useful herbs are chaste tree berry, wild yam cream, natural progesterone cream, St. John's wort, calendula, motherswort, licorice root, black cohosh, dong quai, damiana, sarsaparilla, burdock root, peony root, oatstraw and raspberry leaf.

## Headaches, Depression, Night Sweats And Mood Swings

Some women feel a deep depression, have recurring headaches, fatigue and mood swings with menopause. This could be directly related to hormone changes. On the other hand, these subjective complaints, part of what's called "menopausal syndrome," are sometimes blamed on hot flashes. Other symptoms that fit into menopausal syndrome include fatigue, insomnia, dizziness, palpitations and joint and muscle pains.

After thinking about menopausal syndrome and its connection to hot flashes, it all made sense to me. These symptoms aren't a mystery. If you woke up in the middle of the night on a regular basis drenched in sweat from a hot flash, wouldn't you have insomnia, feel tired and subsequently irritable, nervous and perhaps have headaches? I know I would.

As for menopausal depression, the research done on this symptom may be flawed and results vary from study to study. For example, age, not menopause, is frequently used as a marker in these investigations. A National Institute of Mental Health report showed that women 45 years and older actually suffered less occasions of depression than younger females.[17]

Otherwise, there are nervine herbs, plants that work directly on the nervous system, that can help restore your sense of well being and release stress. Some of these plants are oatstraw, passion flower and St. John's wort. Siberian ginseng is an alternative, often used to soften physical and emotional stress and balance out your body.

Other plants, known more as female healing herbs, include wild yam cream (you can also use natural proges-terone cream), dong quai and chaste tree berry. Dandelion root helps hormonal conditions since it works directly on your liver.

## Bleeding Disorders: Excessive Bleeding And Spotting

A perimenopausal symptom often includes heavy bleeding. It could be caused by build-up of blood-rich tissue if not enough progesterone is produced. It could be a sign of more serious problems such as uterine fibroids, polyps or uterine or cervical cancer. If heavy bleeding last for more than a month, check with your physician.

In the meantime, you can try a low fat diet and avoid dairy for a while to see if it helps. These remedies may be benefical: Wild yam cream, natural progesterone cream, chaste tree berry, yellow dock, sarsaparilla, peony, white oak bark, shepherd's purse, oatstraw, burdock root, nettles, dulse, alfalfa, parsley root, Siberian ginseng, bilberries and cayenne.

## Skin Changes

You may notice the changes in skin tone (not necessarily from baking in the sun) and discover wrinkles as your hormonal lev-els change. Your collagen level declines with age, fine lines appear and wrinkles develop. As androgen hormones are pro-portionately higher, facial hair can result.

These remedies may help: Wild yam cream, natural progesterone cream, licorice, sarsaparilla, sage, chamomile, fennel, dandelion, royal jelly, ginseng and aloe vera.

# Menopausal Wisdom

Most women I have talked to learn about menopause through other women's experiences. You may have mixed emotions and fears regarding aging. Your feelings and attitudes affect not only your hormones, but the way you will experience the transition. I strongly believe that menopause is a natural part of womanhood—a time to be celebrated, not mourned. In many societies, menopause marks the point in a woman's life when she gains a special inner wisdom and a degree of life experience that makes her the respected wise individual of the society. The term "crone" was not originally a negative one, but rather a term of respect, used to describe older women who were highly regarded.

My experience has shown the older women in the United States many times do not do not receive the respect they deserve. Our culture values youth and beauty to such an extraordinary degree that women fear reaching menopause— because they believe it marks the end of their being seen as desirable and valuable, not to mention the end of their fertility. I really applaud the thoughts expressed in Gail Sheehy's book, *The Silent Passage,* where many women finally shared their experience of menopause. What really struck me is that for the very first time, women are realizing that menopause is not a fatal disease or even dangerous. It shouldn't be suffered in silence. Menopause is no longer a road marker that means "This Way to the End." Today, age 50 is the apex of the female life cycle. Finally, the baby boomers are demanding that menopause be more properly seen as the gateway to a second adulthood, a series of stages never before part of the predictable life cycle for other than the very long-lived.[18]

There are many women I have met recently who do find their menopausal years to be ones of positive change. They see their children reach adulthood and leave home at this time. For the first time in many years, they don't have to be mothers—they can take care of themselves and pursue their own dreams. Having the choice to use natural solutions is the best part of that dream.

# Summary

- Menopause is a natural part of womanhood.

- Menopause has four stages during its "transition lane change".

- Decreasing hormonal levels cause menopausal symptoms like hot flashes, night sweats, vaginal dryness, mood swings and insomnia.

- Hysterectomy or artificially induced menopause is an emotional and physical shock to the body.

- Women with hysterectomies often suffer deep depression, hot flashes and many other PMS and menopausal symptoms.

- Natural solutions like wild yam cream, natural progesterone cream, herbs, diet and nutrition give women plenty of choices in managing menopause.

- Menopause is a time of new opportunities and experiences, not an end.

# Chapter 7

# Are Your Shrinking? What About Osteoporosis?

WE COME INTO THIS world as tiny, toothless babies, wearing diapers for the first few years of our lives and we may leave this world in exactly the same way. From Pampers™ to Depends™! From Crest™ to Polident™! Have you ever felt that as we grow from infants to children to adults, this process is reversed as we enter the senior years, including our size? I have discovered the people I know, especially older women, are shrinking! Is this normal? Does bone loss and osteoporosis have to be part of aging?

When I went to the first Holocaust Convention in Washington, D.C., aside from the serious emotional aspects, I couldn't help noticing how short the 10,000 to 15,000 Holocaust survivors were. I didn't even think about osteoporosis at that time. I assumed it was the horrible diets and stresses they had to endure during the war. Now, I realize it was more than war that contributed to their small stature. Osteoporosis is also tied to what's happening with our hormones as we age.

I first noticed my own mother was shrinking when I stood next to her a couple of years ago. All my life, I have looked up to her. Today, it feels like I look straight into her eyes. I am 4 feet 11 inches proud. I would like to say 5 feet tall, but it's just not the truth. I can't afford to get any smaller. I'd have to shop in the children's department! A friend once said to me, "If I water you, will you grow?" Unfortunately I am not a plant. But plants can be part of the solution to osteoporosis. Since natural progesterone is made from the wild yam, it's conceivable wild yam cream could possibly have benefits as well. As we learned in Chapter One, taking the whole plant can have advantages over using just one isolated constituent of an herb. We'll now look at the years beyond menopause and my findings about natural progesterone and natural solutions to your thinning bones.

# What Is Osteoporosis?

Osteoporosis is a condition characterized by a decline in your bone density and thinning of bone tissue, resulting in weak bones prone to fractures. Normally our bodies continually replace old bone tissue with new. When we're children, more tissue is added than removed as bones grow and lengthen. After about age 35, we start to lose the bone replacement war. Gradually, bone mass decreases for both men and women. This is a natural part of aging.

---

### RISK FACTORS FOR OSTEOPOROSIS

1. Stress.
2. Family history of bone disease, especially osteoporosis.
3. Short and thin body type, fair skin.
4. Deficiencies in calcium, magnesium and Vitamin D caused by caffeine intake, alcohol, cigarette smoking and carbonated beverages.
5. Lack of exercise and sedentary lifestyle.
6. Diet high in salt, protein and fat.
7. Declining hormones.
8. Total hysterectomy before age 45.
9. Early menopause.
10. Not having children, or having them late.
11. Kidney or liver disease.
12. Low calcitonin.
13. Diabetes.
14. Hypoglycemia (low blood sugar).

---

Osteoporosis is an exaggerated version of this age-related bone downslide. Women are especially vulnerable to osteoporosis because hormones decline with middle-age. Both estrogen and progesterone diminish as women enter menopause. Falling estrogen levels tip the bone recycling machine in favor of bone breakdown. During the first five years following menopause, women can lose two to eight percent of their vertebral bone. Your body can lose bone mass at a rate of one to three percent per year for the five to ten years following menopause.

---

**PHYSICAL WARNING SIGNS THAT
OSTEOPOROSIS MAY BE AHEAD**

1. Chronic low back pain.
2. Loss of height.
3. Periodontal gum disease.
4. Leg cramps.
5. Joint pain.
6. Rheumatoid arthritis.
7. Tooth loss.
8. Premature gray hair.

---

# What Makes Bones Grow?

Bones are living tissue! Just as a tree grows from a seed, your bones grow from cells. Bones are composed of calcium and protein in varying amounts. Your body remodels bone, a process where new bone tissue is constantly being regenerated to replace the old. From childhood to about age 35, bone cells are produced faster than they are broken down. During those years, healthy bones heal quickly when broken. In the years after menopause, bones are slower to repair.

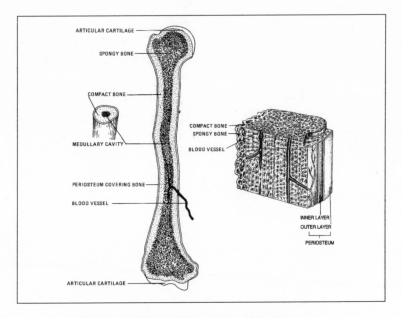

# Meet The Bone's Makers: Osteoblasts And Osteoclasts

Bones are like a concrete wall. Strands of protein called collagen fibers make up the steel beams of your bones. The mineral salts—calcium, phosphate, magnesium, sodium, potassium and carbonate—are the concrete. When your collagen beams are weak, your bones bend easily and become limp like the limbs of a bow-legged child. Without the concrete, especially calcium, your bones become brittle and break easily like in osteoporosis.

Within bone tissue two different types of bone cells exist—osteoclasts and osteoblasts. These cells synchronize their movements to perform the job of recycling your bones by continually replacing old bone tissues with new. New bones can only grow when this bone building activity exceeds the bone dissolving activity.

These cells are especially busy during times of growth or injury. Osteoclasts, very large cells, are set off by the parathyroid hormone and a type of white blood cell called lympho-cytes. Osteoclasts detect older and slightly damaged bone and slowly resorb or dissolve it. Osteoblast cells, on the other hand, are responsible for bringing together the substances needed to form new bone tissue. They fill in the space or hole that is left by the osteoclast and create new bone matter from minerals circulating in your blood.

When these bone demolishing and bone building cells are in balance, bone mass remains stable. However, an overzealous osteoclast or a defect in the bone construction process spurs bone loss.

# Osteoporosis Factors

We really don't know what causes osteoporosis. What we do know is there are many contributing factors. The three most important factors related to bone loss are nutrition, exercise and decline in certain hormones. The loss of estrogen in post-menopausal women causes bone resorption to increase and bone formation to decrease.

Osteoporosis affects both men and women as they age. The United States Department of Health and Human Services estimates that over 20 million Americans are affected by osteo-porosis. The National Institutes of Health reports it affects at least 15 million Americans and is responsible for causing 1.2 million fractures a year. Recent studies have found the United States has the highest rate of bone fractures from osteoporosis in the world. How cheering![1]

## *Lack Of Exercise*

Exercise is beneficial for maintaining healthy bones. The force of impact from regular weight bearing exercise, such as walking, jogging and dancing on the bones helps promote bone growth.[2] One study found that women who walked vigorously four times a week for 50 minutes increased their spinal bone mass by five percent in one year. Non-exercisers lost bone mass at a rate of seven percent a year. To increase walking's advantages, you can wear light ankle and wrist weights.[3]

## Poor Nutrition

Your risk for osteoporosis can be reduced with proper nutrition and by avoiding foods that inhibit calcium absorption. Recent studies have found if your diet is high in fats and sugars, bone strength may lessen and stiffness increase in a relatively short period of time.[4] Diets high in proteins, especially from animal foods like meats, may increase your rate of excretion of calcium in the urine, causing a loss of bone density.[5] A study conducted on women aged 50-64 eating high protein diets (58-92 grams a day), found that even with adequate calcium in the diet, protein still reduced calcium absorption.[6]

## Environmental Pollution

Pollution in our environment, chemicals, food additives and prescription medications contribute to bone loss. Pollution increases your load of heavy metals like lead, cadmium, aluminum and tin, also contributing factors to osteoporosis. Antibiotics, one of the most overused drugs on the market, are not selective when it comes to killing bacteria. While effective in destroying disease-causing bacteria, antibiotics also tend to eradicate the friendly bugs found in your intestine that supply your body with Vitamin K, essential for building bones. Supplementing with lactobacillus acidolphilus and other live cultures found in yogurt and non-pasteurized cultured milk products, can help restore your normal intestinal flora lost from antibiotics. Dairy foods are also high in calcium, which is of course good for your bones.

# Hormones And Shrinking Bones

Hormones play a huge role in preventing you from shrinking and in treating osteoporosis. Why? Women go through hormonal changes from the beginning of peri-menopause to postmenopause. Hormones have a direct effect on your body's ability to build new bone. A proper balance between estrogen and progesterone and healthy thyroid function influence the metabolism of bone matter.

Bone loss starts in your mid-thirties—sometimes estrogen levels decrease at this time, too. Depending on your lifestyle and genetic makeup, this can be the beginnings of osteoporosis. As you age and menopause looms closer, estrogen and progesterone levels decline more, creating a lopsided balance between osteoclasts and osteoblasts activity, in favor of bone degradation. After menopause, the rate of bone loss increases as estrogen levels decrease.[7] Welcome osteoporosis to the stage!

It is also important to look at thyroid function when evaluating osteoporosis. Hyperthyroidism (an overactive thyroid) contributes to high levels of the thyroid hormone thyroxine. Thyroxine maintains proper levels of serum calcium. It also regulates protein, fat and carbohydrate breakdown in all cells. If too high, thyroxine steals calcium from your bones to restore blood levels resulting in thinner bones. Flimsy bones are more prone to fractures. Women taking thyroid medication should be monitored for excess levels of thyroxine, checked for signs of osteoporosis and have bone density tests done.

Low calcitonin, a hormone secreted by both the thyroid and parathyroid glands, has also been found in postmenopausal women with osteoporosis. Since decreased calcitonin may also be implicated in bone loss, scientists have treated osteoporosis with this hormone. So far this hormonal therapy holds much promise.[8]

# Estrogen's Latest Reviews

Early studies of osteoporosis focused mainly on the role estrogen played and how estrogen replacement therapy prevented osteoporosis and heart disease. We're discovering estrogen's affect on our bodies is quite different. The biggest myth surrounding ERT is its failure to prevent and reverse bone loss, as we once thought it did. Over the decades, women using ERT have showed small increases in bone mass and their bone loss was only slowed down.[9]

**Some facts we are now realizing:**

1. Estrogen may decrease the rate of bone resorption.

2. Estrogen minimally retards skeletal mass, but usually does not increase it and bone mass eventually decreases if ERT is stopped.

3. Estrogen facilitates calcium absorption from the intestinal tract and increases parathyroid hormone and calcitonin production.

4. Estrogen may reduce urinary calcium and hydroxyproline excretions which suggest that it inhibits the cells that breakdown bone tissue.

Estrogen is essential in helping your bones to absorb and retain calcium. It also stimulates calcitonin production—which protects your bones. However, oral estrogens reduce the effectiveness and the metabolism of some nutrients necessary for bone health. Also consider that many women who take estrogen supplements experience a delay in bone loss, but not a reversal. Once estrogen therapy is discontinued, bone loss returns to where it would have been without any ERT within five years. Therefore, the benefits of estrogen therapy should be evaluated against the risks before treatment is considered. (See Chapter Three for ERT's side-effects.)

"Estrogen cannot replace bone that has been lost nor straighten curvature of the spine or restore lost height," says Dr. J.D. Gambrell, Jr., "Usually, however it can arrest the disease's progression."[10] New questions are arising on whether estrogen is really necessary for the prevention of osteoporosis—If estrogen fails to build new bones, is it really a necessary ingredient in hormonal replacement therapy? What is progesterone's role, if any, in building new bones?

We need to look at these questions because many doctors haven't considered how these two hormones affect our bones. Perhaps the next generation will have the answers we seek. We know phytoestrogens help boost estrogen activity in menopausal women. We know herbs like chaste tree berry have progesterone-like qualities. Maybe when all the facts are in on the wild yam, we'll learn it has a role in osteoporosis treatment similar to natural progesterone.

# Progesterone: The Bone Builder

Progesterone is a bone-building hormone in its own right. Most early research studies did not consider the role of progesterone in osteoporosis. The failure of estrogen to make new bones led researchers to look at progesterone's function in preventing bone loss. Years before the onset of menopause, your body's production of progesterone begins to decrease, too. Therefore, the decline of progesterone may contribute to loss of bone mass in the years prior to menopause. This can contribute to an increased risk of osteoporosis.

Recent research suggests progesterone plays a role in forming new bone matter, therefore it could help prevent osteoporosis. Experiments with progesterone therapy on female beagle dogs, whose ovaries were removed, showed this hormone binds to osteoblast receptors which in turn increases the rate of bone formation. Progesterone also slows down bone loss in postmenopausal women. Progesterone acts on bone even when estrogen levels are low or absent.

If progesterone works on osteoblasts to increase bone formation, theoretically it could complement estrogens action in decreasing bone resorption. Osteoporosis could actually be a progesterone deficiency disease, not one of low estrogen, because it acts directly on osteoblasts to promote new bone formation.[11] Also, progesterone curbs calcium loss from bones, thereby enhancing bone strength and growth.

Alan Gaby, M.D., author of the book, *Preventing and Reversing Osteoporosis,* and a well recognized authority in nutritional medicine, says, "Preliminary evidence suggests that, in many cases, natural progesterone may be the only hormone needed to prevent or treat osteoporosis and that estrogen replacement therapy may be necessary only to treat hot flashes, postmenopausal depression and vaginal atrophy."[12]

In 1990, Jerilynn Prior, M.D., of the University of British Columbia in Vancouver, Canada indicated progesterone can make new bone tissue. Dr. Prior discovered women athletes who were anovulatory (not ovulating) had low progesterone levels and normal bone mass loss. Dr. Prior observed that nonovulating women with a short luteal phase lost an average of 2.8 to 4 percent of spine bone per year. Remember, progesterone secretion increases during the luteal phase of your menstrual cycle. So a short luteal stage probably means your progesterone levels are lower than normal. Dr. Prior theorized that progesterone stimulates bone formation when she observed women with the lowest blood levels of progesterone showed the greatest degree of bone destruction. Estrogen therapy alone does not guarantee prevention of bone loss as 50 percent of fractures occur in women who are taking estrogen replacement.[13] It is generally accepted that amenorrhea (no period) contributes to osteoporosis too.

# Natural Progesterone Cream In Action

Since 1982, Dr. John Lee has had extraordinary results with natural progesterone cream made from the wild yam in preventing osteoporosis with his postmenopausal patients. He states, "Present osteoporosis management emphasizes prevention rather than cure since true reversal has proven unobtainable by conventional methods. With the hypothesis that progesterone is the missing ingredient for normal bone-building in women, transdermal progesterone cream supplementation (with or without) estrogen was tested in an office based setting over the past six years. Treatment resulted in progressive increases in bone mineral density (BMD) and, what is more important, definite clinical improvement as evidenced by pain relief, height stabilization, increased physical activity and fracture prevention. The benefits achieved were found to be independent of age. It is concluded that osteoporosis reversal is a clinical reality in a program that is safe, uncomplicated and inexpensive."[14]

Dr. Lee's treatment program for osteoporosis is based on his belief that for bones to grow successfully, we need to recreate the conditions under which normal bone building occurs. In his clinical practice, he followed 100 of his patients, ranging in age from 38 to 83. He observed a ten percent increase in bone mass in the first six to 12 months and yearly increases of three to five percent until the bone mass stabilized to that of a healthy 35 year old woman. Some of his patients showed a 20 to 25 percent increase in bone density during the first year.

His treatment program combines diet, nutritional supplements, exercise and a three percent transdermal natural progesterone cream (made from the wild yam) applied daily. He also noticed that supplementation with Vitamin D, calcium and estrogen delayed, but did not reverse, osteoporosis. Fluoride, an experimental and controversial osteoporosis treatment, seemed to increase bone mass, but not strength. The incidence of fractures in non-vertebral bone actually increased with fluoride use.[15]

Dr. Lee's clinical study proved bone mass could increase with progesterone replacement therapy and the damage of osteoporosis could be reversed. The patients with the lowest initial bone densities seemed to progress the quickest. Overall he observed stabilized height, relief from aches and pains, increased mobility and higher energy levels and no side-effects. During this treatment, none of the women suffered from fractures.

---

### DR. JOHN LEE'S OSTEOPOROSIS PREVENTION PROGRAM USING NATURAL PROGESTERONE CREAM

*Nutritional supplements*

Vitamin D (350-400 IU daily).
Vitamin C (2,000 milligram daily).
Beta-carotene (15 milligram day).
Calcium (800-1000 milligram/day, by supplement or in diet).

*Hormone supplements*

Transdermal progesterone, three percent cream applied daily during phasing out (last two weeks) of estrogen use. Dosage should be 1/2 to 1/3 ounces per month. Apply about 1/4 teaspoon of cream on the stomach, inner arm or thighsóany soft, fatty tissue areas of the bodyóat bedtime for two to three weeks each month. You can also use progesterone cream inside the vagina for vaginal dryness. Stop for one week. Never use when menstruating.

*Estrogen supplements*

If needed for vaginal dryness or excessive hot flashes, 0.3 to 0.625 milligrams daily of conjugated estrogen for the same three weeks progesterone is applied.

*Exercise*

Twenty minutes daily.

*Diet*

Vegetable based diet (limit meat to less than three times a week). Also avoid alcohol, cigarettes, or carbonated beverages.

---

# Different Risks—Different Treatments

Osteoporosis treatment is not the same for everyone. It all depends on your risk factors. Dr. Tori Hudson, N.D., a professor at the National College of Naturopathic Medicine in Portland, Oregon, first determines risk factors for osteoporosis and for heart disease before prescribing treatment. She evaluates a patient's risk on a scale of low, middle or high severity based on information she gathers from their medical history, lab tests, physical exam and a bone density test. She examines a women's body type, lifestyle and looks for the following osteoporosis danger signs: sedentary activity level, fair skin and blue eyes, high consumption of alcohol, cigarette smoking, insufficient calcium intake during pregnancy and breast feeding and certain medications or surgeries that encourage bone loss. Once these risk factors are determined, she uses the following stepladder chart to determine treatment.

For Low Risk Patients

1. Diet, exercise and stress management.
2. Nutritional supplementation.
3. Botanicals.

For moderate risk patients, she adds...

4. Natural or semi-natural creams (including natural progesterone and estrogen compounds derived from soy or wild yam).
   For high risk patients, in addition to diet & nutritional supplements, she adds . . .
5. Friendly conventional hormone drugs (e.g. prescribed natural progesterone)
   Or, if needed...
6. Unfriendly drugs (conventional hormonal replacement therapy).

Dr. Hudson finds women who are at low risk for osteoporosis benefit from herbs like licorice, burdock root, dong quai, wild yam, motherwort, sarsaparilla, chaste tree berry, hops and ginseng. For women at moderate risk, she prescribes semi-natural and natural estrogen or natural progesterone. She believes natural progesterone creams made from the wild yam are stronger than the herbs she uses for low risk patients. These herbs have not been proven to protect against bone loss. With these moderate and high risk women, a family history of osteoporosis is often the biggest factor in determining treatment.

For high risk women, Dr. Hudson uses a friendly version of conventional hormonal therapy. She believes natural progesterone compounded at pharmacies is the same or has the same effectiveness as any natural progesterone cream because they all come from the same source—often the wild yam. "I like to err on the side of caution," reports Dr. Hudson. "If someone has a high risk of osteoporosis, I am not going to count on creams or micronized progesterone. I recommend they take a conventional Ortho-est (an estrogen drug). If they have a uterus, I give them natural progesterone to go with it."

You may find some creams erroneously labeled as "wild yam creams" when, in fact, some or all of the active ingredients in these products are natural progesterone. The progesterone preparations sold by pharmacies are a higher concentration than is found in natural progesterone creams available over-the-counter as cosmetics. The USP grade natural progesterone sold in drugstores can only be obtained through a prescription.

## The Thyroid And Bones

Thyroid and those four tiny glands nestled alongside your thyroid (called the parathyroids) play an important role in preventing osteoporosis. The parathyroid hormones' (PTH) role is to maintain proper blood levels of calcium. When calcium levels drop, PTH increases, sometimes robbing your bones of calcium in order to replenish your blood—kind of like robbing Peter to pay Paul. The problem is that this creative calcium banking can thin out your bones. Thyroxine, your thyroid hormone, also removes minerals from your bones to keep serum levels up. Excessive levels of thyroxine, a potential problem with women taking thyroid medication, can cause too much bone depletion.

Lita Lee, Ph.D., stresses it is important to understand that high thyroid function alone does not contribute to bone loss. Low thyroid hormone, or thyroxine, levels can also disrupt bone regrowth by disturbing progesterone production. Raymond Peat, Ph.D., explains that your ovaries need cholesterol, Vitamin A and thyroxine to make progesterone. Thyroxine stimulates the synthesis of cholesterol, the raw material needed to make progesterone and other steroid hormones. So if your thyroid is not functioning at full capacity, there will not be adequate progesterone production. The bottom line, says Dr. Peat, is that your liver and thyroid need to be taken care of for healthy bones. Menopause is a prime time for thyroid problems.

Dr. Peat suggests a list of foods to avoid for women with low thyroid function. He believes simply eliminating these foods alone may bring thyroid hormones up to normal levels. Foods to avoid: All unsaturated vegetable oils, foods in the cabbage and mustard family—especially eaten raw; peanuts, cashews and lentils—because of unsaturated oils and other chemical constituents. Raw cabbage foods and nuts can interfere with iodine's role in thyroxine production, thereby creating low thyroid hormone levels.

Dr. Peat is also a great believer in coconut oil, which he says is "excellent for the thyroid." One to two tablespoons of coconut oil daily added to scrambled eggs or milk shakes, or used instead of butter, and a sluggish thyroid will jump into gear. You may even find you lose weight. Milk and orange juice are also pro-thyroid foods, claims Dr. Peat. Many women, in an attempt to solve their hormonal problems, use treatments that have an anti-thyroid effect. Therapies such as dong quai, evening primrose oil and borage oil should be avoided if you have low thyroid function, advises Dr. Peat.

# Natural Progesterone Versus Progestogens

New combinations of estrogen and progesterone in HRT offer more protection against bone loss than ERT. In addition, for the first time, natural micronized progesterone has been studied with positive results. This new research illustrates that natural progesterone alone appears to be the safest and most beneficial therapy for bone loss with the added ability to build new bone.[16]

As of 1995, estrogen replacement can be supplemented with low doses of oral micronized progesterone to prevent bone loss, promote bone growth and relieve menopausal symptoms. A combination of estradiol with oral micronized progesterone efficiently controls estrogen induced proliferation of the endometrium.[17] Progesterone and progestogens have been found to help prevent osteoporosis by inhibiting calcium loss from bones and promoting growth of bones. Since there are over five different types of progestogens, each kind can have very different results and side-effects.

Joel Hargrove, M.D., of Vanderbilt University Medical Center compared oral micronized natural progesterone to oral progestogens. He discovered that micronized natural progesterone did not give patients the side-effects of increased facial hair, depression, fluid retention, breast tenderness and headaches as did these synthetic progesterones.[18]

Christine Northrup, M.D., recommends natural progesterone cream for women who don't want to use estrogen. She
suggests a program of natural progesterone cream, dietary
changes and exercise. Progesterone dosages are varied
throughout the menstrual cycle, therefore see your doctor
about how you can use progesterone to prevent bone loss.

Dr. Northrup believes women who are not ovulating regularly long before menopause are at a higher risk for bone
loss when they hit menopause. Her healthy bone program is
very similar to Dr. John Lee's, with the addition of a high complex carbohydrate, low-fat diet and low protein. She discour-
ages cola and other carbonated drinks because their high
phosphorous levels interfere with calcium absorption. She
also recommends the following supplementation on a daily
basis.[19]

2000 milligrams of Vitamin C.

300-800 milligrams of magnesium.

1000-1500 milligrams of calcium if you eat a high protein
diet (400 milligrams for a low protein diet).

2-12 milligrams of boron.

350 IU Vitamin D (three minutes in the sun will provide
300-350 units of Vitamin D).

25,000 units beta carotene.

Estrogen can be added for vaginal dryness or hot flashes.

# Prevention With Natural Solutions

## *Natural Medicine—Herbs For Bone Boosting*

Nature's medicine chest contains herbs valuable for safe and
natural healing. Some herbs restore hormonal balance, sup-

port bone growth, improve circulation and supply nutrients needed for bones to grow. To the best of my knowledge, there have not been any scientific studies on herbs' effectiveness in treating osteoporosis, though anecdotal reports from women say they may help. One woman who called me had osteoporosis so badly she was permanently bent over. She was using wild yam cream, along with magnesium and calcium supplements. She excitedly reported to me that her back appeared to be straightening out and her pain was retreating. If you suspect you have osteoporosis or have a strong family history of this disease, check with a qualified practitioner for medical advice. If you would like to try a more natural osteoporosis prevention and treatment program, some of the following tips might help.

## Herbs

I think some herbs help because of the bone-building nutrients they possess and in some cases the way in which they support and heal structures like your muscles and tendon that are in and around the bone. In some instances, they may affect bone healing directly. Helpful herbs for bones are horsetail, dandelion, oatstraw, chaste tree berry, black cohosh, alfalfa, borage seed, licorice root, nettles, dong quai, mustard and kelp. Natural progesterone cream and wild yam cream can be included here, too. Herbs for better blood circulation (and thus healing)—hawthorn, Siberian ginseng, motherwort, bilberries, capsicum and ginkgo biloga. Vitamin E is also helpful.

## Diet

Face it, we are what we eat and what we don't eat. Prevention often lies in our diets. There are many nutritional factors contributing to bone loss. Many of the foods common to the typical American diet are nutritionally depleted before we even bring them home. Many Americans have significant nutritional deficiencies without realizing it. High intakes of caffeine, protein, salt, sugars, soft drinks and processed foods deplete your body of calcium and other important vitamins, minerals and enzymes necessary for healthy bone production. Calcium absorption is also affected by the amount of fat in your diet.

In 1988, The National Women's Health Network found in countries where women ate less calcium than Americans, the incidence of osteoporosis was actually much lower than the women in the United States. The Bantu women of South Africa consume only 220 to 440 mg of calcium each day, yet osteoporosis is rare.[20] It's not enough to eat a lot of calcium to ensure strong bones. You also need to control those substances and habits that rob the body of calcium such as caffeine, alcohol, smoking, sugar, sodium, phosphates and excessive animal protein.

## Coffee And Caffeine

Did you know your morning cup of coffee is robbing your bones? Susan Dawson-Hughes studied 205 healthy, non-smoking postmenopausal women with above average calcium intakes of 774 milligrams daily and a coffee habit of two to three cups a day. She found even this small amount of java stole away calcium. The more coffee you drink and the less calcium you take, the more bone you lose.[21]

## Nutritional Supplements

The supplementation of calcium has been recommended for women since the 1950's to reduce the risk of osteoporosis. Calcium, important for maintaining bone mass and preventing osteoporosis, needs to be supplemented years before menopause begins. Almost all of the calcium you take is deposited in your bones and teeth. The remaining amount is dissolved in your blood and bodily fluids to regulate certain metabolic processes, carry nerve signals to contract muscles, clot blood, keep your heart beating, work with enzymes and help absorb iron.

A deficiency in calcium can cause teeth to decay and bones to break. However, excessive amounts are a problem as well. For example, too much calcium can cause kidney stones in susceptible individuals. When calcium is taken orally, only one third of it is absorbed by your body. The amount of calcium your body keeps depends on the balance between the amount of calcium absorbed by your body and the amount lost each day through your urine. During menopause, lower estrogen levels cause excessive bone turnover, releasing large amounts of calcium into your blood stream, much of which is urinated away.

## BONE NUTRIENTS

| Nutritional Supplements (dietary source) | Role |
|---|---|
| Calcium (Dairy products, dark green leafy vegetables, sardines) | Improved bone mineral density. |
| Phosphorus (meat, yeast, white flour, processed foods) | Improved bone mineral density. |
| Magnesium (lean meat, whole grains, seeds) | Needed for connective tissue, cartilage, bones. |
| Zinc (whole grains, seeds, lean meat) | Improved collagen and bone. |
| Manganese (beans, lean meats, liver) | Reduces bone breakdown |
| Copper (liver, whole grains) | Strengthens tissues and bones. |
| Vitamin C (citrus fruit, green vegetables) | Needed to make collagen. |
| Vitamin D (cereals, cheese, eggs) | Assists calcium absorption. |
| Vitamin K (green leafy plants) | Aids in synthesis of protein and absorption of calcium. |
| Boron (fruits, vegetables) | Assists in calcium absorption and increases estrogen levels. |

Like any part of your body, bones need a wide range of nutrients—not just calcium—to stay healthy. Phosphorus, magnesium, manganese, zinc, copper, silicon, enzymes and Vitamins A, C and K are high on that list. These vitamins and minerals enjoy a complex working relationship—where proper amounts of each is necessary for the others' absorption and function in your body. That's why it's best to get your nutrients from high quality foods. If you think you're still lacking, try a good multiple vitamin/mineral supplement containing an appropriate balance of vitamins and minerals.

Your bone's collagen fibers require Vitamins A and C. Vitamin D and hydrochloric acid in the stomach help absorb calcium. As we age, hydrochloric acid, an acidic substance vital for the absorption of calcium and other nutrients, decreases. This is one reason why some older people are low in certain minerals and vitamins. Absorption of vitamins is an important factor in osteoporosis. There's no point taking supplements if your body can't use the nutrients.

Phosphorus is essential to all soft tissue, as well as bones and teeth. Calcium even needs phosphorus to be metabolized. However, phosphorus is a tricky mineral. Too little phosphorus can cause brittle bones and inhibit bone growth. Too much phosphorus, common in our American diets full of meat and soda pop, depletes calcium from your bones.

---

## MEDICATIONS THAT INTERFERE WITH CALCIUM ABSORPTION

**Corticosteroids**—Suppress new bone formation.
Cortisone, Hydrocortisone, Prednisone, Dexamethasone

**Anti-convulsants**—Stimulate production of enzymes, breaks down of Vitamin D, leading to calcium and Vitamin D deficiencies.
Phenytoin, Phenobarbital, Primidone, Phensuximide.

**Antacids containing aluminum**—Increase calcium excretion.

**Diuretics**—Increase calcium excretion.

---

# How Magnesium Works

While magnesium and calcium have similar functions, they are rivals. Calcium contracts muscles, magnesium relaxes muscles. Whereas calcium may induce kidney stones, magnesium tends to prevent them. Too much magnesium inhibits bone calcification while excessive calcium can cause magnesium deficiency. The trick is take enough of each of these minerals in the right amounts. Doctors have been arguing for years about what an appropriate ratio of calcium to magnesium should be—two to one, one to one or one to two. What we do know is many of the same factors that rob your body of calcium—like alcohol and too much protein—do the same to magnesium.

About 60 percent of magnesium in your body is in the bones. A recent study published in the Journal of Applied Nutrition showed an increase in bone density in post-menopausal women who took more magnesium and less calcium. Magnesium suppresses the secretion of the parathyroid hormone, PTH, which regulates the levels of calcium in bones and soft tissues. "The PTH draws calcium out of the bones and deposits it in the soft tissues, while calcitonin increases calcium in the bones."[22] This process must have the proper amount of magnesium or this chemical action won't occur. Magnesium also helps your body use B vitamins, vital for estrogen utilization. Peanuts, bran, lentils, tofu, wild rice, bean sprouts and chicken are all good sources of magnesium.

Wild yam and natural progesterone are, in essence, kissing cousins. The natural progesterone used to successfully treat and prevent osteoporosis is made from the wild yam. So it makes sense that wild yam may also have a role in osteoporosis treatment.

# Summary

- Prevention is the key to osteoporosis treatment.

- Change your diet.

- Progesterone can build new bones.

- Estrogen slows down bone loss.

- Natural progesterone cream helps prevent and reverse bone loss.

- Herbs may help.

- Exercise regularly.

- Vitamins C & D, magnesium, calcium, boron and beta-carotene help keep your bones healthy.

*Part Three*

# THE LIGHT
# AT THE END
# OF THE
# TUNNEL

# Chapter 8

# YOU SPEAK TO ME! MAPPING YOUR OWN JOURNEY

OVER THE YEARS THAT I have been researching and lecturing about natural solutions, women have shared their stories with me. You are not the only woman living with terrible symptoms like monthly cramps, or bloating, or mood swings, or gaining weight, or always feeling tired, or depressed, or craving chocolate, or breaking out in acne or having a hot flash, or night sweats...

This chapter is a place for women to learn from one another—to tell their stories about success with natural solutions—especially with the wild yam and natural progesterone. You do have choices! Read on...

## *Leslie's Discovery: Hysterectomy induced menopause at age 30*

After my hysterectomy, I went into a very deep, long depression. I was unaware of the emotional problems I would encounter after my surgery. I didn't feel like a total woman. I lost interest in my life. I no longer went out socially or had an interest in being with friends. I felt that no one really understood what it felt like to lose my reproductive organs and the ability to have children at age

30. I was young and unprepared for this loss. I truly suffered emotionally for years. Each time I saw a child, a deep pain went through my heart. My doctor immediately prescribed hormone replacement therapy. I started with shots of Premarin (a synthetic estrogen). I continued to try other estrogen drugs, finally settling on a tolerated form of replacement therapy, the Estraderm patch.

For almost ten years I had noticed loss of hair, weight gain, severe migraines, stomach problems, loss of sex drive, and increasingly poor vision that declined to the point where I was declared legally blind without my glasses. I never talked to my gynecologist about the problems I was experiencing, but rather I called an internist or an eye doctor or my family doc about each individual problem. Although my internist knew I was taking hormones, he prescribed various drugs to relieve my headaches and other problems. The system of treatment I experienced was one of taking drugs to counteract the drugs. None of my doctors tried to backtrack to find the original problem.

My sister told me how the wild yam cream helped her PMS depression. I was reluctant to do anything without my Doctor's approval. When I called my gynecologist to ask him about it, he did not have any knowledge about natural therapies. He told me that I would be on hormones until the day I died. I was scared, and just accepted what he said, following his treatment unquestioningly.

At first, I used both therapies for months. I finally I had enough faith in the wild yam cream to go off the estrogen patch. Gradually, I went off the patch, first changing it once a week, then every two weeks, every month, and finally discontinued its use At the same time, I was using the wild yam cream every morning and evening. Since I have stopped using the patch, and began using wild yam cream with natural progesterone, my symptoms have decreased. I lost 20 pounds within two months of discontinuing the synthetic hormones. My appetite returned to normal, and my hair stopped falling out. I didn't realize until I stopped using the patch how much the drugs had caused me discomfort all these years. I practically had a personality change. During the time I was using the patch, I had attributed all my symptoms to other causes. Now, I am know it was the side effects of estrogen replacement therapy. Today, I look and feel like I did before my hysterectomy. I realized the benefits of natural progesterone when I was going through artificial menopause and hope every woman can experience the release and relief that I have.

## Holly's Story: Stress induced PMS

Holly was going through a difficult and intense divorce. She was unaware she was suffering from PMS. Her primary physicians regarded her symptoms as something that was in her head and "just due to stress." He prescribed Valium. The first two weeks of the cycle, Holly felt okay. Beginning with ovulation, she began to notice headaches and slight mood swings. The week before her period, she felt more and more depressed, hopeless, and nervous. The day before her period, she felt like crawling out of her skin, crying, moody, and rode an emotional rollercoaster. Life became unbearable. Every month she felt a deep hopeless depression and anxiety. Life became unbearable. At times, she even had thoughts of suicide. She felt bloated, had breast tenderness, and severe cramps. Unfortunately, the prescription of Valium as a stress reliever didn't help these problems. After three months with no results on the Valium, she stopped taking all the pills. She heard that wild yam cream helps for relieve depression and menstrual problems. She found a wild yam cream with chaste tree berry and apricot kernel oil and began to use it as a facial moisturizer for two weeks before her period. In just one cycle, Holly noticed her symptoms were reduced, by the fourth cycle, she was happier that she had been in years and free from depression and the PMS symptoms (and free from her unsympathetic husband, too)!

## *Sheila Admits: Miscarriage*

Sheila is a 25-year old hairdresser who suffered a miscarriage in her third month. For the first time in her life, she found herself feeling too depressed to even get out of bed. She couldn't ever remember feeling this way before—she was usually a positive, energetic person. After her miscarriage she began to feel very negative about her life and her marriage, and was experiencing dramatic mood swings. She wasn't even sure if she wanted to have a family anymore. She felt as if her whole life had changed. What she didn't know was depression is very common after a miscarriage, but her physician did not offer her this information. Then she began using wild yam cream and began to feel much better within four weeks. Sheila's moods stabilized, and she began to feel more positive about her life.

## *Jennifer's Story: No period for three years*

Jennifer was 18 years old when she heard about wild yam cream from a friend. She hadn't gotten her period since she was 15 years old, and had been to many doctors, and had tried the gamut of hormonal treatments. Nothing helped her. She was unhappy, moody, and had developed a terrible temper. After using 1/4 to 1/2 teaspoon of wild yam cream for 27 days, she got her period after three years of absence. Her body finally felt in balance, and her emotional and mental state improved. She felt great—like her old self again.

## *Jill Reveals: Hot flashes*

"I was having severe hot flashes frequently and night sweats for several months. It was interrupting my ability to work, sleep and became very uncomfortable. I first felt my whole face turn red. I become all wet and sweaty. My clothes were wet. I even get heart palpitations. I found myself asking, Is it hot in here, or is it me? I began using a 1/4 - 1/2 teaspoon wild yam cream, twice a day for two weeks it 'got rid' of my problem within a few days."

## *Julie's Story: Vaginal dryness*

She was suffering from vaginal dryness and sex became irritating and unpleasant. Her chiropractor recommended wild yam cream, for her irritation. She began using 1/8 teaspoon of wild yam cream before sex and she was able to relieve the vaginal dryness and enjoy sex once again.

## *Clare's Success: Combination of herbal extracts worked to relieve menopausal symptoms*

She had tried a variety of extracts from a holistic doctor for two months with no relief from emotional menopausal symptoms like anxiety, lightheadedness, and fatigue. Clare tried wild yam cream combined with  other herbs  and in less than a week her symptoms were gone and she felt normal again.

## *Pamela's Surprise: Skin problems*

"I have gone to many doctors this past year to find out what is wrong with my skin. I used wild yam cream, and the next day, my skin problem disappeared."

## *Janis Admits: Night sweats*

"I used wild yam cream for two days and my night sweats disappeared! I rubbed it into my elbow. I am very happy with the results."

## *Etta Says:*

"I had been bleeding excessively for weeks. I was a wits end. I did not want to operate or take synthetic drugs. I wanted to try something natural before I resorted to drugs or surgery. I heard from other women about the wild yam. Once I was able to find a wild yam creme, I used it heavily over my stomach and inner thighs. I about 24 to 36 hours my bleedings stopped. I was so happy to be able have success without drug therapy."

# *Write Your Own Story Here*

# Chapter 9

# WISE WOMAN WITHIN

WITHIN EACH OF YOU is the power to create, nurture yourself and heal. I came to understand how true this is one remarkable August afternoon. I was sitting at my desk and telling a friend on the phone how extraordinarily happy I felt. My usual companions—Grumpy and Weepy—had been replaced with inner peace and joy. I was so content that I began to worry. Perhaps my menopause had arrived early and I would never menstruate again, or have the chance to bear a child. To my surprise, my period quietly began later that day, but without my "normal" premenstrual agony and fanfare.

I was totally stumped by this dramatic change in my health. Then it hit me—it was the wild yam cream I'd been using for four months. This wonderful cream changed the way I felt and looked. I restored my inner balance and beauty. I gained emotional tranquillity. What my Mom couldn't tell me about women's health and hormones, Mother Nature did herself by leading me to natural medicine and the wild yam.

I wrote this book for you—think of it as your gift to wellness. Each page is one mile of the journey I took to find answers and regain my health. Countless conversations with many types of health practitioners, long hours reading the latest research, and plenty of soul searching have allowed me to bring you valuable information.

Along my journey of discovery, I identified the love-hate relationship between progesterone and estrogen. I learned the benefits of wild yam and natural progesterone cream, how hormones work in your body, and where natural medicine can fit into your health regimen.

Most importantly, I listened to women like you who shared their experiences with wild yam cream to end PMS, reduce their hot flashes and wipe away menopausal problems. Wedged between their words, I heard joy and excitement about the safe and effective alternatives they found to Hormone Replacement Therapy (HRT).

On this last mile of my journey with you, I want to share my most important discovery of all. YOU DO HAVE A CHOICE. You can choose your health care, and as I found out, you can choose to be healthy or not. It may take longer using natural therapies. It may take additional time to pinpoint the exact road you need to find your own inner peace. Fortunately, the time spent on this gift of health is well worth it.

Let me share one last tale with you. I heard an inspiring fable about a little girl and a snake. One day, this young child was walking in the forest and was about to cross a creek when a snake appeared. "Please little girl," he pleaded, "please pick me up and carry me across the creek." The little girl replied, "No, Mr. Snake, I won't. If I do, you'll bite me." The snake promised he wouldn't bite her. In fact, he said so repeatedly, begging the girl to carry him over the body of water. Finally, the little girl gave in and picked him up. As she was traveling across the creek, the snake bit her. In her astonishment, she screamed, "Mr. Snake, you bit me! You promised you wouldn't do that!" The snake looked her straight in the eye and quietly said, "You knew what I was when you picked me up."

To me, this story illustrates that knowledge isn't often enough. True wisdom comes from acting upon what you know to be true—using your intuition and listening to that persistent voice inside. By sharing all that I have learned, I hope each one of you makes your own choices. Keep your eyes open and your ears alert to the wisdom that dwells within you. You have the power to take control of your hormones, your health and everything else on your path. Have a wonderful journey!

# *Appendix A:*

# GLOSSARY OF TERMS

**Adrenal cortex**: outer part of the adrenal gland that secretes steroid hormones including cortisone-like hormones, the sex hormones estrogen and testosterone, and mineral corticoids like aldosterone responsible for regulating blood pressure. DHEA is also secreted by the cortex.

**Adrenal glands**: small pyramid-shaped glands that sit on top of each of the two kidneys and secrete hormones.

**Adrenal medulla**: the inner part of the adrenal gland that secretes epinephrine (adrenaline) and norepinephrine. These hormones are released in response to stress.

**Amenorrhea**: failure to menstruate.

**Amino acids**: the basic building blocks required for the formation of proteins. Some amino acids can be produced by the body, while the essential amino acids are only obtained from foods.

**Androgen**: a generic term for an agent, usually a hormone, that stimulates male-like qualities.

**Androstenedione**: a weak androgen abundantly secreted by the ovaries, adrenal glands and testes. It is a major source of estrogen after menopause.

**Anovulatory cycle**: menstrual cycle without ovulation or the release of an egg.

**Antioxidant**: substance that prevents oxidation or inhibits damaging free radical reactions promoted by oxygen. Many nutrients are antioxidants such as vitamins E and C, and flavonoids in plants and food.

**Atrophy**: a loss or wasting of size of a part of the body.

**Basal metabolic rate (BMR)**: the lowest, waking metabolism or heat production of an individual at the lowest level of cell chemistry. One way to record the BMR is to take your temperature upon waking in the morning before doing anything else. To take your BMR temperature you should have fasted all night, be at complete physical and mental rest and be lying in a moderately warm room.

**Beta carotene**: also called pro-vitamin A. A yellow-red pigment found in plants, like carrots and yams, that the body converts into vitamin A. Also an antioxidant nutrient.

**Bioflavonoids**: substances found in fruits and plants essential for the absorption and processing of vitamin C. They are needed to maintain collagen and may protect against infection.

**Blood sugar**: amount of glucose or sugar circulating in the bloodstream.

**Calcitonin**: hormone made by the parathyroid and thyroid glands. It guards the body against high blood levels of calcium and phosphorus. Because calcitonin inhibits osteoclast activity (bone breakdown), it prevents calcium loss from the bones.

**Cervix**: part of the uterus that extends into the vagina.

**Cholesterol**: fat-like substance found in animal-based foods and made in the body. Cholesterol is the raw material for steroid hormones.

**Collagen**: the main protein comprising the bone, connective tissue and cartilage.

**Corpus luteum**: literally means "yellow body." This body is the remnant after a follicle in the ovary releases its mature egg (during ovulation). The corpus luteum secretes progesterone and some estrogen.

**Corticosteroids**: steroid hormones produced by the adrenal glands or cortisone-like drugs that resemble the adrenal glands' glucocorticosteroid hormones.

**Creams**: a fatty or oil-based substance that may contain healing or moisturizing ingredients like herbs.

**Cysteine**: sulfur-containing amino acid.

**Decoctions**: a type of medicinal tea whereby woody plant parts are simmered in water to dissolve their water soluble constituents.

**Diuretic**: a drug or other substance that promotes urination.

**DNA (deoxyribonucleic acid)**: the fundamental component of living matter. DNA is found in chromosomes and contains information about an animal or plant's genetic code.

**Dysmenorrhea**: painful and difficult menstruation.

**Edema**: swelling. Excessive accumulation of fluid in tissues or cells.

**Endocrine glands**: glands that manufacture hormones and release them into the bloodstream. Included are the adrenal glands, ovaries, testes, thyroid glands, parathyroid glands, pituitary, pineal gland, thymus and pancreas.

**Endometriosis**: a serious condition in which the endometrium (lining of the uterus) grows outside of the uterus. While sometimes without symptoms, this ailment often causes pain, severe menstrual cramps and perhaps infertility.

**Enkephalin**: a pain relieving substance found in the brain.

**Enzyme**: protein secreted by cells to speed up specific bio-chemical reactions.

**Estradiol**: the most potent naturally occurring estrogen.

**Estriol**: a weaker form of estrogen.

**Estrogen**: a group of steroid hormones found in both men and women. It is responsible for the development and mainte-nance of female characteristics and reproductive functions in women.

**Estrone**: a form of estrogen.

**Fibrocystic breast disease**: lumps in the breast that increase and decrease with a woman's menstrual cycle.

**Fibroids**: noncancerous fibrous (composed of fibers) growths commonly found in or on the uterus wall.

**Fluid extract**: a liquid containing concentrated amounts of medicinal herbs.

**Follicle**: a small, round sac in the ovary containing an egg.

**Follicle stimulating hormone (FSH)**: a hormone released by the pituitary that stimulates the growth and maturation of fol-licles in the ovaries.

**Free radicals**: highly reactive molecules possessing an unpaired electron; damage cells and tissues in the body.

**Glucose**: a simple sugar. Carbohydrates from food are usually converted into glucose for transport in the bloodstream.

**Glucose tolerance factor (GTF)**: a chromium-containing com-pound that aids insulin in the control of blood sugar.

**Glycogen**: a major carbohydrate made from glucose. It is stored mainly in the liver and muscles until needed for energy and other body functions.

**Hemoglobin**: a complex protein found in the blood that contains iron and carries oxygen from the lungs to the tissues.

**High density lipoprotein (HDL)**: the smallest lipoprotein in the blood which carries cholesterol and fats from cells to the liver. HDL cholesterol is also known as the "good" cholesterol.

**Homeostasis**: the body's natural state of equilibrium with respect to various functions and chemical compositions.

**Hormone**: a chemical substance produced in one part of the body that has specific effects on another part.

**Hypoglycemia**: low blood sugar.

**Infusion**: a medicinal tea in which the tender parts of plants, such as leaves and flowers, are briefly soaked in freshly boiled water to withdraw the herb's water soluble constituents.

**Lipoprotein**: compounds that contain both protein and fat.

**Lotions**: water/oil based solutions used for either cosmetics or as medicines.

**Low density lipoprotein (LDL)**: a protein that carries cholesterol and fats throughout the blood. LDL cholesterol is also known as the "bad" cholesterol.

**Luteinizing hormone (LH)**: a hormone produced by the pituitary gland that stimulates the follicles in the ovaries to mature and release their eggs, and to secrete progesterone.

**Menorrhagia**: abnormally heavy menstrual bleeding.

**Metabolism**: the transformation in the body of the chemical energy of foodstuffs to mechanical energy or heat.

**Metrorrhagia**: any irregular bleeding from the uterus between periods.

**Natural progesterone**: this term refers to progesterone made from the wild yam, soybeans and sometimes animal sources. Natural progesterone is a regulated chemical called USP grade progesterone. According to what many experts have told me, natural progesterone is identical in structure to the progesterone found in your body.

**Ovary**: one of the pair of female reproductive organs which produces an egg, and the hormones estrogen and progesterone.

**Ovulation**: the release of an egg from an ovary about two weeks before menstruation begins.

**Pancreas**: an organ with both endocrine and digestive functions. The pancreas secretes digestive juices into the intestinal tract containing enzymes that break down protein, fat and carbohydrates. The endocrine portion of the pancreas secretes insulin and glucagon directly into the blood to control blood sugar levels.

**Phytohormones**: refers to "plant hormones." This term is inaccurate since plants don't contain hormones per se, only animals do. This label usually refers to constituents with hormone-like activity like phytoestrogens (compounds with estrogen-like action). These compounds exert a very weak effect on the body compared to naturally occurring and synthetic hormones.

**Pituitary gland**: found in the brain, this structure is called the master gland because its hormones control other endocrine glands in the body.

**Precursors**: usually a physiologically inactive substance that is converted into an active chemical substance like an enzyme, vitamin or hormone.

**Progesterone**: a female sex hormone produced by the ovaries mainly during the second half of the menstrual cycle. It helps promote the growth of the uterine lining and maintains pregnancy. Progesterone is also released by the placenta during pregnancy, and by the adrenal glands.

**Progestins**: a generic term for any substance, natural or synthetic, that exerts a progesterone-like effect. Progesterone, natural progesterone and progestogen all fit into this category.

**Progestional**: this adjective merely describes any substance (usually progesterone or a progesterone-like drug) that helps maintain pregnancy in a woman.

**Progestogen**: this is a synthetic drug that has some progesterone-like effects. Progestogens are usually made from natural progesterone. That is, the starting materials for progestogens are also wild yam and soybeans, but progestogens are more processed than natural progesterone.

**Prostaglandins**: one of several hormone-like fatty acids that act on several organs affecting the circulatory, nervous, and reproductive systems and metabolism.

**Testosterone**: a male sex hormone, found in both males and females, which induces masculine characteristics and supports a man's reproductive organs.

**Thyroid gland**: an endocrine gland responsible for regulating the rate of metabolism.

**Tinctures**: solutions of either alcohol, vinegar or glycerine that contain medicinal herbs.

**Uterus**: the womb in a female.

**Vagina**: forms a canal to the cervix in a female.

# *Appendix B:*

# An Easy to Read Vitamin & Mineral Chart & Symptoms of Nutrient Deficiencies

EVERY WOMAN I KNOW needs to know the truth about vitamins and minerals and nutrients. You've heard all the claims about a mineral or how great Vitamin E is for your nails, but is that information all in one place and easy to find? This is an alphabetical chart that doesn't just describe the benefits of these wonderful natural solutions. Here, you can discover how they function in your body, the signs of nutrient deficiency, the foods and herbs containing them and what situations and substances will deplete your body of nutrients.

I've also included for your safety, toxicity signs for each nutrient. It's easier to overload on some nutrients, especially the fat-soluble vitamins like Vitamins A, D and E. If, while taking these nutrients, you experience any of these toxicity signs, stop taking those nutrients immediately. To be perfectly safe, check with your nutritionally-wise practitioner before taking any nutrient for a longer time or in large amounts.

# Vitamins

## *Vitamin A*

Essential for growth and maintenance of healthy skin, bones, teeth, hair, nails and eyes. Needed for proper functioning of the immune system. Involved in healing wounds. Important for health, reproductive and adrenal gland function. Involved in thyroxine formation.

***Conditions that may be helped:*** PMS, osteoarthritis and rheumatoid arthritis. Prevents night blindness, irregular periods, fatigue, vaginal dryness, dry skin, endometriosis, fibrocystic breast disease, acne, Crohn's disease, gastric ulcers.

***Depleted by:*** Heat, processing foods, coffee, low-fat diet, ERT, alcohol, cortisone, mineral oil, fluorescent lights, lack of protein.

***Deficiency signs:*** Night blindness, defective tooth enamel, retarded growth, impaired bone formation, decreased thyroxine formation.

***Toxicity signs:*** May produce toxicity in large amounts. Nausea, vomiting, headache, blurred vision, dizziness, lack of coordination, loss of appetite, weakness, rash, itching, fatigue, weight loss, irritability.

***Food sources:*** Dairy products, eggs, yellow and dark green vegetables and fruits such as carrots, sweet potatoes, squash, broccoli and cabbage; also fish oils, liver.

***Herbal sources:*** Peppermint, alfalfa, raspberry, dandelion greens, kelp, cayenne, paprika, sage, black cohosh, rose hips.

## *Vitamin B complex*

Important for healthy digestion, liver function, emotional stability, anxiety, hot flashes and the heart. Vitamin B complex is actually ten water soluble vitamins, not stored in the body, that have interrelated functions. B vitamins are useful for promoting liver function. If there are insufficient levels of Vitamin B complex, it affects estrogen levels.

***Conditions that may be helped:*** High blood pressure and fatigue.
***Depleted by:*** Tobacco, sugar, alcohol, coffee, estrogen replacement therapy (ERT).

***Food sources:*** Whole grains, liver, carrots, molasses, fruits, fish.

***Herbal sources:*** Oatstraw, red clover, parsley.

The following is a list of the individual vitamins that are part of the B-complex family.

## Vitamin B-1 (thiamine)

Essential for development and growth, a healthy nervous system, muscles, bones, blood vessels, teeth and gums. Helps with the absorption of iron, and improves appetite. Converts carbohydrate foods into energy. Normalizes metabolism of estrogen and other hormones. Involved in synthesis of fatty acids, acetylcholine and the nucleic acids RNA and DNA.

***Conditions that may be helped:*** Depression, apathy, anxiety.

***Depleted by:*** Excess sugar intake, stress, sulfa drugs, cigarettes, coffee, tea, alcohol, dieting, illness, surgery, ERT, heat.

***Deficiency signs:*** Easily fatigued, loss of appetite, irritability, emotional instability, confusion, loss of memory, stomach pain, constipation.

***Toxicity signs:*** Headaches and irritability.

***Food sources:*** Wheat Germ, liver, whole grains, legumes, oatmeal, peanuts, brown rice, fish, beans, sunflower seeds.

*Herbal sources*: Alfalfa, burdock, catnip, briar rose buds, rose hips, peppermint, yellow dock, fenugreek, raspberry leaves, nettles.

## Vitamin B-2 (riboflavin)

Essential for transforming proteins, fats and carbohydrates into energy. Needed for building tissues and protecting against skin, eye, nail and hair disorders. Aids in the formation of antibodies and helps prevent sensitivity to light in the eyes. Important for the synthesis of corticosteroid hormones, red blood cells, and the co-enzyme active forms of Vitamin B-6 and folic acid.

*Conditions that may be helped*: EEG abnormalities, eye problems.

*Depleted by*: Coffee, sulfa drugs, stress, ERT, sunlight, antibiotics, alcohol, junk foods.

*Deficiency signs*: Cracks and sores in the corners of the mouth, red, sore tongue, burning eyes, sensitivity to light, apathetic, dizzy, vaginal itching, oily skin.

*Toxicity signs*: No known toxicity.

*Food sources*: Dairy products, liver, whole grains, green vegetables such as brussels sprouts, peas, nuts, sunflower and sesame seeds, red meats, yogurt, chicken, brewers yeast, seaweed, spirulina.

*Herbal sources*: Alfalfa, fenugreek, rose hips, nettles, yellow dock, hops, peppermint, parsley, echinacea, ginseng.

## Vitamin B-3 (niacin, niacinamide, nicotinamide, nicotinic acid)

Energy production for over 100 enzymes. Important for the

conversion of food into energy. Improves circulation and reduces cholesterol. Essential for healthy skin, gums and digestive tissues. Aids nervous system function.

***Conditions that may be helped:*** Osteoarthritis and rheumatoid arthritis.

***Depleted by:*** Alcohol, coffee, stress, antibiotics, sugar, sulfa drugs, sleeping pills, ERT.

***Deficiency signs:*** Muscular weakness, fatigue, loss of appetite, indigestion, rashes, insomnia, bad breath, nausea, vomiting, recurring headaches, tender gums, deep depression.

***Toxicity signs:*** When you first take niacin, you'll experience what's called a "niacin flush": red face and upper body, itching, stomach upset. This reaction is not harmful, except perhaps in people with peptic ulcers or asthma. Chronic toxicity signs include liver damage, increased uric acid in blood and impaired glucose tolerance.

***Food sources:*** Chicken, fish, peanuts, legumes, broccoli, squash seeds, cashews, peas, beans, avocado, brewer's yeast, mushrooms, whole grains.

***Herbal sources:*** Alfalfa, hops, raspberry leaf, red clover, echinacea, licorice, rose hips, parsley.

## *Vitamin B-5 (pantothenic acid)*

Essential for the metabolism of food and release of energy for cellular function. Vital for formation and synthesis of hormones and support of the adrenal glands.

***Conditions that may be helped:*** Osteoarthritis and rheumatoid arthritis. Fatigue, restlessness, irritability, depression, neuritis, decreased coordination.

***Deficiency signs:*** Deficiency is rare.

*Toxicity signs:* Rare.

*Food sources:* Liver, eggs, nuts, legumes, whole grains.

## Vitamin B-6 (pyridoxine)

Essential for metabolism of amino acids, healthy teeth, gums, red blood cells and nervous system. Regulates brain activity and growth. Aids in the synthesis of neurotransmitters and utilization of DNA and RNA needed for the process of cell reproduction. Important for metabolism of hormones and immune function.

*Conditions that may be helped:* PMS symptoms such as water retention and irritability. Osteoarthritis and rheumatoid arthritis. Combats nausea and vomiting associated with pregnancy. Convulsions, depression, lack of muscle coordination, carpal tunnel syndrome.

*Depleted by:* Alcohol, coffee, stress, heat, sunlight, high protein diet, sugar, cortisone, penicillin, ERT.

*Deficiency signs:* Low blood sugar, hair loss, cracks around mouth and eyes, numbness and cramps in arms and legs, visual disturbances.

*Toxicity signs:* Losing sense of touch, numb feet, unsteady gait, loss of coordination.

*Food sources:* Chicken, fish, meat, whole grains, eggs, brown rice, liver, banana, sunflower seeds, alfalfa sprouts, wheat germ, prunes, avocado, grapes, peas.

## Vitamin B-12 (cyanocobalamin)

Essential for healthy red blood cells, and proper functioning of all cells, bone marrow, nervous system and intestines. Involved in metabolism of food and synthesis of DNA and RNA.

**Conditions that may be helped:** Low blood sugar, difficulty with concentration, memory loss, depression, agitation, manic behavior, hallucinations, osteoarthritis, osteoporosis, bursitis, some forms of anemia.

**Deficiency signs:** Anemia, neuritis, fatigue, nerve damage, soreness or weakness of arms and legs, decreased sensory perception.

**Toxicity signs:** No known toxicity.

**Food sources:** Dairy products, fish, liver, kidney, milk, meat.

## Biotin

One of the B-complex vitamins. Essential for metabolism of food: amino acids, fatty acids, and nucleic acid. Essential for chemical systems in the body.

**Conditions that may be helped:** Enhances the immune response for Chronic Fatigue Syndrome and candida (yeast) infections. Seborrhea dermatitis, diabetes.

**Deficiency signs:** Depression, lassitude, sleepiness, skin disorders.

**Toxicity signs:** No known toxicity.

**Food sources:** Liver, kidney beans, lima beans, dark green leafy vegetables.

## Choline

Considered one of the B-complex vitamins. It functions with inositol as part of lecithin. Synthesis of phospholipids in the brain and nervous system. Precursor of acetylcholine; involved in nerve transmission. Prevents fats from building up in the liver; helps move fats into the cells. Also essential for healthy kidneys and gallbladder.

**Conditions that may be helped:** Atherosclerosis, hepatitis, high cholesterol, stroke, multiple sclerosis, hyperthyroidism, hypertension, asthma, eczema, alcoholism.

**Depleted by:** Too little protein in the diet.

**Deficiency signs:** Fatty deposits in the liver, heart trouble, bleeding stomach ulcers, bleeding kidneys, high blood pressure, atherosclerosis, hardening of the arteries.

**Toxicity signs:** Long-term, high doses of choline may create a Vitamin B-6 deficiency.

**Food sources:** Liver, whole grains, soybeans, legumes, egg yolk, brewer's yeast, wheat germ; also lecithin.

## Folic acid (folacin)

Another member of the B-complex family. Involved in the synthesis of the nucleic acids DNA and RNA, thus essential for growth and reproduction. Formation of healthy red blood cells. Stimulates production of hydrochloric acid in the stomach and stimulates the appetite. Helps liver function and important for healthy brain function and mental well being.

**Conditions that may be helped:** Pernicious anemia, fatigue, heart disease, prevention of birth defects, adrenal exhaustion, baldness, atherosclerosis, diverticulitis, arthritis, psoriasis.

**Depleted by:** Alcohol, caffeine, sugar, stress, heat, sunlight, oxygen, sulfa drugs, ERT.

**Deficiency signs:** Graying hair, poor growth, swollen tongue, anemia, forgetfulness, sores at mouth corners.

**Toxicity signs:** No known toxicity in most people.

**Food sources:** Green leafy vegetables, spinach, liver, meat, whole grains.

*Herbal sources:* Alfalfa, chickweed, sage, parsley, nettles.

### Inositol

A lipotropic nutrient that is part of B-complex, and similar to biotin and choline. Involved in phospholipid synthesis. Aids in nerve transmission and regulates enzyme activity.

*Conditions that may be helped:* Atherosclerosis, high blood pressure, schizophrenia, glaucoma, baldness, cirrhosis, asthma, insomnia.

*Depleted by:* Coffee.

*Deficiency signs:* Constipation, eczema, hair loss.

*Toxicity signs:* No known toxicity.

*Food sources:* Fruits, grains, vegetables, nuts, legumes, organ meats.

## Vitamin C (ascorbic acid)

This is a primary water-soluble and antioxidant vitamin. It is essential for tissue growth and repair, and formation of collagen. It helps increase the absorption and effectiveness of iron and calcium, and the utilization of folic acid. Involved in the synthesis of neurotransmitters and cholesterol regulation.

*Conditions that may be helped:* PMS and menopausal symptoms. Osteoarthritis and rheumatoid arthritis. Reduces allergic response and relieves pain. Fatigue. Helps with low blood sugar. Enhances immunity by increasing the production of leukocytes—the white blood cells that fight germs. Excessive bleeding, builds stronger bones, heals wounds. High blood pressure.

*Depleted by:* Cigarettes, pollution, stress, antibiotics, aspirin and pain relievers.

*Deficiency signs*: Bleeding gums, tendency to bruise, nose-bleeds, lowered resistance to infections, slow wound healing; if severe—scurvy.

*Toxicity signs*: No known toxicity. However, high doses may interfere with some laboratory tests, reduce fertility in women, cause temporary diarrhea and stomach cramps and decrease copper absorption.

*Food sources*: Fresh fruit and vegetables.

*Herbal sources*: Rose hips, raspberry leaf, parsley, cayenne, paprika, echinacea, skullcap, nettles, dandelion greens, alfalfa, yellow dock roots, hops.

## *Vitamin D*

Promotes calcium absorption and utilization of phosphorous in building and maintaining strong teeth and bones. Induces synthesis of proteins that transport calcium. Maintains blood calcium levels.

*Conditions that may be helped*: Osteoporosis, adult-onset diabetes, fractures, eye problems, gallstones, arthritis, allergies, canker sores, vaginitis.

*Depleted by*: Anti-convulsing medications, cortisone, mineral oil, smog.

*Deficiency signs*: Rickets in children, osteoporosis of long bones, tetany (muscular tingling, spasm and numbness), near-sightedness.

*Toxicity signs*: Kidney and aorta damage, headaches, nausea, diarrhea.

*Food sources*: Liver, milk, tuna, butter, fatty fish, organ meats, liver oil, egg yolks; also direct sunlight.

*Herbal sources*: Not found in plants.

# Vitamin E (tocopherol)

This fat-soluble vitamin is a powerful antioxidant essential for immune function. Lecithin or a meal containing fat or protein help Vitamin E absorption. Selenium operates together with Vitamin E. Essential for the function of red blood cells, and protection of essential fatty acids. Vitamin E, along with Vitamins B1 and B6, iodine, and proper thyroid function, prolactin, dopamine, and prostaglandins inhibit oxidation and facilitate reduction processes that benefit estradiol. Hormone normalizing and stabilizing effects. Acts as a mild prostaglandin inhibitor.

*Conditions that may be helped*: PMS and menopausal symptoms (such as hot flashes), menstrual cramps, cancer prevention, arthritis, wrinkles and other signs of aging. Osteoarthritis and rheumatoid arthritis. Fibrocystic breast disease. Nervousness, fatigue, insomnia, dizziness, heart palpitations, shortness of breath.

*Depleted by*: Excess consumption of polyunsaturated oil, mineral oil, chlorine, heat, freezing, thyroid hormone, sulfates, ERT, milling of grains (removing fiber, bran and germ).

*Deficiency signs*: Muscular wasting, reduced pituitary and adrenal gland functioning, liver and kidney damage, gastrointestinal disease, anemia, infertility, heart disease. Low levels of Vitamin E result in an increase in FSH and LH levels.

*Toxicity signs*: No known toxicity. However, high blood pressure patients and those with chronic rheumatic heart disease should avoid Vitamin E except under expert supervision.

*Food sources*: Vegetable oils, wheat germ, meat, egg yolk, soybeans, green vegetables, whole milk, whole grains, nuts, sunflower seeds, watercress.

*Herbal sources*: Alfalfa, nettles, seaweed, dong quai, dandelion, rose hips.

## *Vitamin K (phylloquinone)*

There are three forms of Vitamin K; two of these (K1 and K2) are made by bacteria in the gut. K3 is a synthetic version. Needed for the synthesis of blood-clotting factors that helps control bleeding. Also important for liver function.

*Depleted by:* Radiation, air pollution, frozen foods, antibiotics, aspirin.

*Deficiency signs:* Hemorrhages, nosebleeds, diarrhea, miscarriages.

*Toxicity signs:* No known toxicity for natural Vitamin K. Synthetic Vitamin K can produce jaundice, flushing, chest constriction and sweating.

*Food sources:* Green leafy vegetables, yogurt, egg yolk, molasses.

*Herbal sources:* Alfalfa, kelp, green tea.

# Minerals

## *Boron*

Essential for bones and strength.

*Conditions that may be helped:* Osteoporosis, menopausal symptoms.

*Deficiency signs:* Depressed growth.

*Toxicity signs:* Stomach upset, nausea, vomiting, diarrhea, rash, lethargy; chronic-signs of osteoporosis.

*Food sources:* Vegetables, fruits and nuts.

*Herbal sources:* Chickweed, purslane, nettles, dandelion, yellow dock.

# Calcium

As the most abundant mineral in your body, calcium is essential for the strength and growth of bones and teeth. It's also involved in the synthesis and regulation of hormones. Calcium activates enzymes that release energy and assists in blood clotting. Along with phosphorous and magnesium, it is vital for heart function.

*Conditions that may be helped*: PMS and menopausal symptoms including bloating, nervousness and insomnia. Menstrual cramps, osteoporosis, high blood pressure.

*Depleted by*: Antibiotics, cigarettes, high protein diet, sugar, fat, inactivity, alcohol.

*Deficiency signs*: Muscle cramps, numbness and tingling in the legs and arms, joint pains, tooth decay, insomnia, irritability; extreme and long-term deficiency causes osteoporosis.

*Toxicity signs*: Excess calcium can be deposited in the soft tissues and form kidney stones.

*Food sources*: Sardines, almonds, dairy products, salmon, tofu, broccoli, beans, molasses, sunflower seeds, peas, kale.

*Herbal sources*: Valerian, kelp, nettles, horsetail, peppermint, oatstraw, parsley, raspberry leaf, borage, dandelion leaf.

# Chlorine

This is an electrolyte that helps maintain body fluid and acid/alkaline balance. Stimulates hydrochloric acid production in the stomach. Chlorine helps with hormone distribution, liver function and keeping joints healthy.

*Conditions that may be helped*: Diarrhea, vomiting.

*Deficiency signs*: Hair and tooth loss, poor digestion and muscle contraction.

*Food sources:* Seafood, seaweed, salt.

# Chromium

This mineral is important in the metabolism of food, activation, and regulation of cholesterol. It is a cofactor of glucose tolerance factor (GTF), which helps insulin's regulation of glucose.

*Conditions that may be helped:* Fatigue, diabetes, hypoglycemia, heart disease.

*Depleted by:* White sugar, refining of food.

*Deficiency signs:* Depressed growth, severe glucose intolerance in diabetics.

*Toxicity signs:* No known toxicity for dietary chromium.

*Food sources:* The most absorbable forms are brewer's yeast (which contains the chromium compound called glucose tolerance factor GTF), liver, beef, beets, molasses from beet sugar, mushrooms and whole wheat bread.

*Herbal sources:* Licorice, echinacea, sarsaparilla, wild yam, oatstraw, yarrow, valerian root.

# Copper

Important for immune function and energy metabolism. Copper plays an important part in the formation of hemoglobin and red blood cells, and glucose and cholesterol metabolism. Involved in the synthesis of collagen and elastin together with Vitamin C. Cardiovascular function, as well as the skeleton, central nervous system and thyroid all rely on copper.

*Conditions that may be helped:* Osteoporosis, excessive bleeding, water retention, arthritis, anemia, heart arrhythmia.

**Deficiency signs:** Relatively unknown. Weakness, skin sores.

**Toxicity signs:** Nausea, vomiting. Copper intake over 3.5 grams can be lethal.

**Food sources:** Green leafy vegetables, seaweed, nuts, grains, liver, almonds.

**Herbal sources:** Sage, horsetail, skullcap.

# Iodine

Essential for the synthesis of thyroxine, a thyroid hormone that controls metabolism and influences estrogen and other hormones. Iodine is important in promoting growth and development, and regulating energy production. Vitamins A and zinc are needed for iodine metabolism. Needed for healthy, hair, skin and nails.

**Conditions that may be helped:** Fatigue, fibrocystic breast disease, thyroid and liver function. Low blood sugar. Deficiency or inability to metabolize iodine results in enlargement of the thyroid gland (goiter) or hypothyroidism.

**Deficiency signs:** Goiter, hypothyroidism, dry hair, rapid pulse, heart palpitations, nervousness.

**Toxicity signs:** No known signs from food and water sources of iodine. Iodine in medicines can impair thyroid hormone synthesis in a person with normal thyroid function.

**Food sources:** Iodized salt is the most important source of iodine. Also seaweed and seafood.

**Herbal sources:** Sarsaparilla, kelp, parsley, celery.

# Iron

Combines with protein and copper to make hemoglobin,

which transports oxygen within the red blood cells throughout the body. Important in immune function, thyroid function and metabolism of food. Needed for beautiful skin.

*Conditions that may be helped*: Hot flashes, excessive bleeding, insomnia, night sweats, fatigue, light-headedness, headaches, iron-deficiency anemia.

*Depleted by*: Coffee, tea, alcohol, carbonated drinks, high altitude, excess dairy, blood loss. Tannic acid, phytic acid and phosphates decrease absorption.

*Deficiency signs*: Most common sign is anemia which includes the following symptoms: difficulty breathing, brittle nails, constipation, fatigue.

*Toxicity signs*: Heart problems, internal bleeding, kidney and liver problems, death.

**NOTE**: Never take iron supplements unless you know you're deficient or you're advised to take them by your physician. Therapeutic doses of iron can cause constipation, and may increase your risk of heart disease, cancer and diabetes.

*Food sources*: Liver, wheat bran, pistachios, sunflower seeds, dried apricots, molasses, almonds, raisins, tofu, turkey, haddock, spinach, pumpkin seeds, cashews, lima beans, soybeans, peanuts, sprouts, peas, brewer's yeast.

*Herbal sources*: Dandelion root, burdock, catnip, kelp, dong quai, black cohosh, sarsaparilla, licorice, nettles, kelp, chickweed.

## Magnesium

This mineral is required by over 300 enzymes for energy metabolism. Magnesium is also involved in body temperature control, making protein from amino acids and transporting messages through nerves to the muscles. Together with calcium, phosphorous, Vitamin D and other nutrients, magnesium helps keep bones healthy.

**Conditions that may be helped**: Osteoporosis, PMS and menopausal symptoms, diabetes, fatigue, weakness, irritability, sleep problems, high cholesterol, high blood pressure, headaches.

**Depleted by**: Alcohol, phytic acid in whole grains, large quantities of fluoride or zinc, diuretics, ERT; refining foods removes magnesium.

**Deficiency signs**: Tremors, confusion, irregular heartbeat, depression, irritability.

**Toxicity signs**: No known toxicity (unless you have kidney disease or possibly certain types of bone tumors or cancers).

**Food sources**: Peanuts, lentils, split peas, tofu, wheat germ, banana, oatmeal, wild rice, bean sprouts, almonds, chicken, spinach, beef, salmon, nuts.

**Herbal sources**: Licorice, kelp, nettles, horsetail, oatstraw, evening primrose.

## *Manganese*

Important for synthesis of fatty acids, cholesterol and for formation of bone, blood and collagen. Activates enzymes. Manganese feeds the brain and nervous system, and is essential for the production of sex hormones and thyroxine.

**Conditions that may be helped**: Diabetes, fatigue, epilepsy, multiple sclerosis, allergies, asthma, schizophrenia.

**Depleted by**: Chemical fertilizers, processing and milling of food.

**Deficiency signs**: Ear noises, dizziness, loss of hearing, decreased glucose tolerance; may trigger seizures in epileptics.

*Toxicity signs:* No known toxicity for dietary forms, although very high amounts may impair iron utilization. Industrial exposure to manganese can result in the toxic signs of weakness, impotency, and irritability.

*Food sources:* Seaweed, whole grains, egg yolks, nuts, seeds, green vegetables.

*Herbal sources:* Raspberry leaf, uva ursi, ginseng, wild yam, hops, catnip, echinacea, kelp, nettles, dandelion.

## *Phosphorus*

Important for strong bones and teeth, and kidney and nerve function. Plays a role in metabolic energy production and activation of B vitamins. Vital for niacin and riboflavin digestion.

*Conditions that may be helped:* Osteoporosis, atherosclerosis, arthritis, stress.

*Depleted by:* Antacids.

*Deficiency signs:* Decreased appetite, weight loss, overweight, fatigue and irregular breathing.

*Toxicity signs:* No known toxicity (except in cases of kidney disease).

*Food sources:* Nuts, seeds, whole grains, fish, meat, eggs, poultry.

*Herbal sources:* Peppermint, yellow dock, fennel, hops, chickweed, nettles.

## *Potassium*

A primary electrolyte important for cells, regulating and controlling fluids, water and acid based (pH) balance inside cells. Important in regulating heartbeat. Influences muscular contractions and cramping.

**Conditions that may be helped:** Water retention, fatigue, high blood pressure, stroke, polio, mononucleosis, fracture.

**Depleted by:** Alcohol, coffee, sugar, stress, fasting, diuretics, laxatives, high salt intake.

**Deficiency signs:** Insomnia, constipation, general weakness, poor reflexes, acne, dry skin.

**Food sources:** Vegetables, fruits, whole grains, sunflower seeds.

**Herbal sources:** Peppermint, sage, catnip, hops, dulse.

## Selenium

Selenium is an antioxidant and protects your body from free radical damage, and ensures enough oxygen for energy producing cells. It preserves tissue elasticity. May play a role in the metabolism of antioxidants like Vitamin E. Prostaglandin synthesis relies on selenium.

**Conditions that may be helped:** Angina, hypertension, stroke, cystic fibrosis, arthritis, infertility.

**Depleted by:** Chemical fertilizers, acid rain, processing and cooking foods, refining grains. Low selenium levels in soils affects selenium content in foods grown there.

**Deficiency signs:** Premature aging.

**Toxicity signs:** Hair loss, fingernail changes, nausea, abdominal pain, fatigue, irritability, diarrhea, peripheral neuropathy.

**Food sources:** Lobster, tuna, shrimp, ham, eggs, chicken, whole grains, breads, dairy products, cereals.

**Herbal sources:** Black cohosh, valerian, echinacea, kelp, ginseng, hawthorn berries, fenugreek, sarsaparilla, uva ursi.

# Zinc

Required by over 100 enzymes that make DNA for cell replacement and protein synthesis from amino acids. Releases energy from glucose and fats. Makes hydrochloric acid in the stomach which is important for digestion. Involved in the production of sex hormones and thyroid hormone synthesis. Aids in the formation of collagen, a component of connective tissue.

*Conditions that may be helped*: PMS and menopausal symptoms, diabetes, osteoarthritis, rheumatoid arthritis, high blood pressure, heavy periods, skin conditions such as acne and eczema, combats effects of aging.

*Depleted by*: Alcohol, ERT, stress, infection.

*Deficiency signs*: Stretch marks, white spots in the fingernails, brittle hair and nails, poor wound healing, irregular menstrual cycles.

*Toxicity signs*: Nausea, diarrhea, vomiting, stomach upset. Therapeutic use of zinc should be restricted to six months, unless given by a nutritional practitioner, as zinc interferes with copper metabolism.

*Food sources*: Oysters, nuts, cashews, turkey, fish, wheat germ.

*Herbal sources*: Wild yam, chickweed, echinacea, nettles, sarsaparilla, skullcap, sage.

# Other Nutrients

## Bioflavonoids

Bioflavonoids work together with Vitamin C. This group of compounds protects connective tissues, and controls bruising and internal bleeding.

*Conditions that may be helped*: Osteoarthritis, rheumatoid

arthritis, menopausal symptoms such as hot flashes and night sweats, hemorrhaging, premenstrual breast and water retention, anxiety, herpes of the mouth.

**Food sources:** Citrus fruits.

**Herbal sources:** Buckwheat greens, hawthorn fruits, rose hips, horsetail, blue green algae, elder berries.

## Essential fatty acids

Essential Fatty Acids (EFA's) are not made in the body, for example linoleic acid. EFA's are vital as prostaglandin building blocks (precursors) that contribute to control and function of organs. EFA's help lubricate hair and skin, prevent dry skin and hair loss.

**Conditions that may be helped:** PMS and menopausal symptoms, osteoarthritis, rheumatoid arthritis, heavy periods.

**Food sources:** Nuts and seeds like flax, pumpkin, sesame, sunflower or wheat germ oil.

**Herbal sources:** All wild plants contains some EFA's. Borage oil, black currant seed oil, flaxseed oil, evening primrose oil.

## Glucosamine sulfate

Important for joint repair, and protects against joint destruction. It aids in the manufacturing of cartilage components.

**Conditions that may be helped:** Osteoarthritis and rheumatoid arthritis.

**Food sources:** Lobster, crabs and mussels.

# Symptoms Of Nutrient Deficiencies Table

| SYMPTOMS: | DEFICIENCY MAY BE FROM: |
|---|---|
| **General** | |
| Cold feet and hands | Iodine |
| Loss of taste | Zinc |
| Insomnia | D, Calcium, Magnesium |
| Poor dream recall | B-6 |
| Excess ear wax | B-complex, Choline and Inositol |
| Low energy | B-complex, Iodine, Iron |
| Nervousness | B-complex, Calcium and Magnesium |
| Varicose veins | C, E, Iron, Copper |
| **Cardiovascular** | |
| Elevated blood pressure | Choline, Calcium, Potassium, Selenium, Chromium |
| Slow or irregular heartbeat | B-complex, Potassium |
| Muscle weakness | D, B-5, Calcium, Potassium |
| **Respiratory System** | |
| Prone to infections | A, B-complex, C, Potassium |
| Sinus problems | A, B-complex, C, Potassium, Zinc |
| Dryness | A, D, E, Zinc |

| Symptoms: | Deficiency May Be From: |
|---|---|
| **Gastrointestinal System**<br>(*Note:* **Many of these symptoms can also indicate a nutrient toxicity.**) | |
| Bloating and gas | B-complex, Zinc |
| Nausea | A, B-3, B-6, Magnesium |
| Infrequent hard bowel movements | Iron, Fiber |
| **Hair** | |
| Dandruff | B |
| Dermatitis | B, Essentials Fatty Acids, Zinc |
| Dull, dry | Protein |
| Oily | Choline |
| Thin hair | B, Essential Fatty Acids, Protein |
| Hair grows poorly | Protein, Zinc |
| Split ends | Protein, Zinc |
| **Skin** | |
| Brown pigmentation | B, C, E |
| Bruises easily | C, K |
| Dry and flaky | A, B, E, Essential Fatty Acids |
| Stretch marks | B, E, Zinc |
| White pale skin | B, C, Iron |
| Protruding veins | Bioflavonoids, C, Zinc |
| Slow healing wounds | C, Zinc |
| Scaly, rough arms | A |
| Yellowish coloring | B-6, Choline, Magnesium |
| Oily skin | B-6 and B-complex, Choline and Inositol |

| SYMPTOMS: | DEFICIENCY MAY BE FROM: |
|---|---|
| **Mouth** ||
| Bad breath | B-complex, B-3, Zinc |
| Canker sores | A, B-complex, Zinc |
| Cracks on lip corners | B-1, B-2, and B-3 |
| **Tongue** ||
| Green color | B-complex, B-6, Choline |
| White color | B-complex, C, Choline |
| Magenta coating | B-complex, B-12, Potassium |
| Thick white spots | A, B-complex |
| Scalloped sides | B-6, B-12, Folic acid |
| **Gums and Teeth** ||
| Cavities | B-complex, Calcium, Zinc |
| Grinding teeth | Calcium, Magnesium |
| Periodontal disease | Calcium |
| **Nails** ||
| Brittle | Iron, Calcium, Protein, Essential Fatty Acids |
| White spots | Zinc, Calcium |
| Spoon-shaped | Iron, Zinc |

# *Appendix C:*

# HERBAL MATERIA MEDICA

THIS MATERIA MEDICA FOCUSES on herbs helpful for women's reproductive conditions. Some of the herbs listed below contain phytoestrogens and other hormone-like compounds that help correct hormonal imbalances. These plants are winners for your health and beauty because they work on many levels at the same time. I list the English or common name first, then the Latin name so you know exactly what you should be using.

While these herbs are wonderful medicines, they should only be taken at the appropriate times and in the correct amounts for specific conditions. Don't take herbs "just because." Sometimes medicinal herbs are contraindicated (shouldn't be taken) if you have a particular condition or are taking certain medications. A nursing or pregnant woman should never take herbs or anything else before talking to her physician. If you want to try herbs for a health problem, consult with a qualified herbalist or physician versed in herbalism first.

## Alfalfa                              (*Medicago sativa*)

Alfalfa is a valuable nutritive herb with a high mineral and vitamin content; rich in beta-carotene, Vitamins C, D, E, K and B, calcium, phosphorus and potassium chlorophyll, protein, as well as phytoestrogens. It is useful for treating menopausal symptoms, arthritis, as a mild diuretic, to counteract internal bleeding from ulcers, reduces blood sugar levels, lowers blood cholesterol, aids in indigestion and prevents tooth decay. It can be applied externally to aid wound healing.

Research studies with monkeys, rats, and rabbits on high cholesterol diets showed alfalfa saponins lower cholesterol levels. Alfalfa also has an estrogenic effect on grazing animals and helps improve general health and vitality.

## Angelica                  (*Angelica archangelica*)

This plant is useful for stimulating the appetite and improving assimilation of food, relieving inflammatory conditions such as bronchitis, and helping pleurisy and pneumonia. It is a soothing aid for menstrual cramps, intestinal colic and poor digestion. If taken in large amounts, it will first stimulate, then paralyze the central nervous system. The species *Angelica sinesis,* contains phytoestrogens helpful in conditions characterized by both high estrogen (some types of PMS) and low estrogen (menopause). (*See also* Dong quai)

## Bilberry                  (*Vaccinium myrtillus*)

Bilberry is rich in flavonoids, carotenes, Vitamins A and C, explaining why it helps stabilize collagen and acts as an antioxidant. It has been effective in the treatment of circulatory disorders, night blindness, anemia, diarrhea, controlling blood sugar levels for diabetes, varicose veins and arterial disorders. Also used for blood problems, hemorrhaging, bleeding gums and troubles with blood vessels such as capillary fragility, arteriosclerosis and advanced diabetic vascular complications.

## Black cohosh            (*Cimicifuga racemosa*)

Studies have shown that black cohosh can lower luteinizing hormone and that it contains substances that bind to the estrogen receptors of a rat's uterusóboth of these pieces of research suggest this herb contains estrogenic activity. Black cohosh relieves hot flashes, sleep disturbances, menstrual cramps, muscle spasms, eases childbirth and is a mild sedative for reducing irritability. It can lower high blood pressure and cholesterol levels, and is effective in the acute stage of rheumatoid arthritis and sciatica.

## Black haw                    (*Viburnum prunifolium*)

Black haw is used to treat menstrual cramps, and for threatened miscarriages. Its antispasmodic and sedative properties make it useful for some sexual disorders and nervous tension. The uncooked fruit of this plant is *poisonous.*

## Blue cohosh                  (*Caulophyllum thalictroides*)

Blue cohosh is used to treat uterine conditions, such as threatened miscarriages in the last trimester of pregnancy. Also can weakly induce sweating.

## Borage                       (*Borago officinalis*)

This is a source of GLA for prostaglandin formation explaining its anti-inflammatory actions. This is an herb for restoring, supporting and balancing the adrenal glands. It is a diuretic and is said to stimulate flow of milk in nursing mothers. Most of these effects are primarily nutritive.

## False Unicorn                (*Chamaelirium luteum*)

This plant is a uterine and ovarian tonic used to delay menses and relieve ovarian pain. It eases vomiting in pregnancy and helps prevent threatened miscarriage.

## Chaste tree berry     (*Vitex agnus castus*)

The active constituents of this plant have progesterone-like action. Studies in Germany showed extracts of *Vitex* stimulated the release of luteinizing hormone and inhibited the release of follicle stimulating hormone. *Vitex* stimulates and normalizes pituitary function. It can help regulate female hormonal imbalance, and reduce menopausal and PMS symptoms. *Vitex* is used for amenorrhea, endometriosis, irregular menstrual cycles, menstrual cramps, uterine fibroids, menopausal symptoms such as hot flashes and dizziness and premenstrual water retention. It is used throughout Europe for PMS and menopause as a natural solution to hormone replacement therapy.

## Cramp bark     (*Viburnum opulus*)

This plant is a sedative and strong antispasmodic useful for menstrual cramps, irregular menstrual periods and miscarriages.

**WARNING**: the fresh berries are *poisonous*.

## Dandelion root     (*Taraxacum officinale*)

Dandelion is rich in various nutrients such as potassium, and Vitamins A and D. Its high choline levels feed the liver. Dandelion aids both liver and gallbladder function, important in the handling of estrogen and other hormones. It is a blood cleanser, diuretic, a mild laxative, aids in weight loss and helps with the absorption of calcium which can strengthen bones, thus preventing osteoporosis.

## Dong quai     (*Angelica sinensis*)

It is this species of *angelica* that contains phytoestrogens. Dong quai is an important female remedy in Chinese medicine for hormone regulation. It is used for PMS, menstrual problems and menopausal symptoms. It is said to alleviate fatigue and cramping, lower blood pressure, helps anemia, pain and swelling, and protects the liver. It acts as a sedative and immune stimulator.

**CAUTION**: Do not use during menstruation.

## Evening primrose          (*Oenothera biennis*)

This GLA-rich herb affects prostaglandin production. It can be used for the control of PMS, infertility, post-menopausal problems and skin conditions. Evening primrose is expected to have a direct effect on the liver.

## Fenugreek          (*Trigonella foenum-graecum*)

This plant is rich in protein, EFAs, lecithin and phytosterols. Fenugreek has been used to help balance blood sugar, nourish glands, control cellulite, improve digestion and increase libido. It is said to promote fertility, and soothe upset stomachs and the uterus and promote lactation.

## Ginger          (*Zingiber officinale*)

This pungent spice is most famous for its antinausea affects during motion sickness and the nausea and vomiting of pregnancy. As a pain reliever, ginger can also reduce menstrual cramps.

## Ginseng          (*Panax ginseng*)

This supposed cure-all is claimed to be a "sexual rejuvenator." In animal studies, ginseng has accelerated ovarian growth and enhanced ovulation. The active ingredients in ginseng, called ginsenosides, exert estrogen-like activity on the vagina, enough to prevent vaginal dryness during menopause.

Ginseng has also been shown to fight both mental and physical stress, stimulate immunity, support the liver (important for hormone balance), treat diabetes and have anti-aging effects.

There are so many adulterated ginseng products on the market, therefore it's difficult to assess whether ginseng has any adverse effects. However, those who've taken large amounts of ginseng or taken ginseng for extended periods of time have occasionally reported hypertension, euphoria, nervousness, insomnia, skin rashes and morning diarrhea. If you experience any of these, discontinue using ginseng. When you continue again use for two weeks on and two weeks off.

## Hawthorn berry (*Cratagus oxycantha*)

I included this cardiac herb because a woman's chance of developing heart problems increases dramatically after menopause. This herb is rich in flavonoids which can help to open coronary blood vessels. It can alleviate hypertension and reduce angina attacks. Hawthorn berry is used for irregular heartbeats, nervous disorders, insomnia and coronary artery and other vascular disorders.

## Kelp (*Fucus vesiculosus*)

This seaweed is an important general nutritive tonic essential for proper hormone regulation and menstrual problems related to low thyroid function. Kelp is rich in iodine, chromium and other minerals, with antibiotic and thyroid stimulating activity. It helps supply iodine to the thyroid, useful in cases of hypothyroidism. If low thyroid function is a problem, kelp may improve skin texture and dull hair, help burn excess fat and enhance metabolism. It can be used externally for arthritic joints.

**CAUTION**: Be careful to take kelp only if you have a true iodine deficiency, as too much of this herb may cause thyrotoxicosis and heart damage.

## Licorice root    (*Glycyrrhiza glabra*)

This well-recognized hormone balancer contains isoflavones that are believed to possess estrogen-like activity, useful for balancing female hormones. Research showed nonovulating women given licorice root extract began ovulating again. The glycyrrhetinic acid in licorice protects the liver against chemical damage and its glycyrrhizin may help hepatitis. Licorice root can be taken for peptic ulcers, canker sores, colds, bacterial infections, allergies, inflammatory problems, menstrual problems and menopausal symptoms such as hot flashes. It's reported to strongly support adrenal gland function.

**CAUTION**: Because licorice has aldosterone-like affects, it probably shouldn't be used by people with a history of high blood pressure, kidney failure or current digitalis use. If you use licorice for a long time, have your doctor monitor your blood pressure and electrolytes, and make sure you're consuming enough potassium.

## Motherwort    (*Leonuus cardiaca*)

As an emmenagogue (an agent that increases menstrual flow), motherwort is good for cases of amenorrhea (no menstrual period). It also helps menstrual cramps. Motherwort has been used as a menopausal herb for hot flashes, night sweats, emotional mood swings, to strengthen the heart, reduce anxiety and as an antispasmodic. It eases false labor pains.

**CAUTION**: Using this herb may cause contact dermatitis.

## Nettle    (*Urtica dioica*)

Nettles are a rich source of trace elements. It is used for eczema, hay fever, sinusitis, anemia, exhaustion, wound healing, menstruation, menopausal problems and externally for arthritis. Nettle acts like a mild diuretic, may lower blood sugar, is a laxative and helps stop bleeding.

### Raspberry leaf       (*Rubus idaeus*)

The leaf of the raspberry plant is a good all-over herb for women's problems during menstruation, menopause, pregnancy and delivery. It helps ease painful menstrual flow, menorrhagia, relieves nausea during pregnancy and relaxes uterine muscles. Although raspberry leaf is generally accepted as safe during pregnancy, as with all herbs check with your practitioner before taking anything.

### Sarsaparilla root       (*Smilax sarsaparailla*)

This herb is most famous for its tonic and blood cleansing abilities. Sarsaparilla seems especially adept at binding endotoxins, bacterial byproducts that can aggravate inflammatory conditions like arthritis, gout and psoriasis. Because of its widespread tonic effects, sarsaparilla has been used for infertility, menopausal hot flashes, vaginal or uterine infections, menstrual problems and skin conditions. Although some manufacturers claim this herb contains testosterone, this is highly unlikely.

### Saw palmetto berry       (*Serenoa repens*)

Known primarily as an herb for helping an enlarged prostate in men, saw palmetto has also been give to women to prevent shrinking of ovaries, the vagina, breasts and bladder. It contains fatty acids and phytosterols which have been shown to inhibit the conversion and binding of testosterone to receptors, thus blocking testosterone's action and promoting its breakdown. Based on this information, saw palmetto may also benefit female conditions where there is too much androgen hormone, such as in polycystic ovarian disease.

Saw palmetto has also been reported to help menstrual problems and cramps, urinary tract disorders, diabetes, infertility, thyroid deficiency and low sex drive, increase lactation, act as a mild sedative for the nervous system, stimulate appetite, aid digestion, and help hot flashes, vaginal-uterine infections, and rheumatism.

## Squaw vine berry (*Mitchella repens*)

This herb is useful for relief of painful menstruation and to prepare for childbirth. It is a uterine tonic, and improves digestion as well. Again, check with your practitioner before using this or any other herb during pregnancy.

## Wild yam root (*Dioscorea villosa*)

Wild yam actually refers to 150 or more species. This plant contains plant sterols used to make progesterone and other steroid hormones in the laboratory. It is unknown at this time whether the human body can convert these sterols into hormones. Although there is no scientific proof as of yet, many users claim that wild yam root cream helps combat menopausal symptoms and other female conditions related to hormonal imbalance.

Traditionally, wild yam root has been used to treat menstrual cramps, and ovarian and uterine pains, arthritis, intestinal colic, soothe diverticulitis, liver troubles, bilious colic, muscle pains, problems of childbirth, calm nerves, depression, flatulence and indigestion. Wild yam helps incontinence by restoring tone to the bladder. See Chapter Four for more specifics.

## Yarrow (*Achillea millefolium*)

The antispasmodic and anti-inflammatory effects of yarrow make it useful for menstrual cramping. This herb also possesses diaphoretic (sweat-inducing) and fever reducing properties, as well as the ability to lower blood pressure and help with diarrhea.

# *Appendix D*

# REFERENCES

## *Chapter One Notes*

1  Goldberg, B. *Alternative Medicine: The Definitive Guide.*
   Puyallup, Washington: Future Medicine Publishing,
   Inc.,1993, 254.

2  Pizzorno, J. & Murray, M. *A Textbook of Natural Medicine.*
   Seattle, Washington: Bastyr College Publications, 1985.

3  Zenni, M.K. et al. "Streptococcus pneumoniae colonization
   in the young child: Association with otitis media and resistance to penicillin." *Journal of Pediatrics* (1995): 127:533-37.

4  Nikiforuk, A. "Antibiotic arsenal is rapidly being depleted."
   *The Globe and Mail* 21 October 1995, D8.

## *Chapter Three Notes*

1  Gaby, A., M.D., *Preventing and Reversing Osteoporosis.* Rocklin,
   California: Prima Publishing, 1994, 275.

2  Peat, R., Ph.D. Telephone interview conducted by author,
   Minneapolis, March 1995.

3  Lark, S. *PMS: Premenstural Syndrome Self Help Book.* Berkeley,
   California: Celestial Arts Publishing, 1984, 27-28.

4  Follingstad, A.H. "Estriol, the forgotten estrogen?" *Journal of
   the American Medical Association* (1978): 239(1): 29-30.

5  Prior, J., M.D. "Progesterone and the prevention of osteoporosis." *Canadian Journal of OB/Gyn Women's Health Center*
   (1993):1(4):179-81.

6  Lark, S. *PMS: Premenstural Syndrome Self Help Book.* Berkeley,
   California: Celestial Arts Publishing, 1984, 27-28.

7  Budoff, P.W. *No More Hot Flashes*. New York, New York: Warner Books, 1984, 7.

8  *New England Journal of Medicine*, 328:13.

9  Lee, J.R., M.D. *Natural Progesterone. The Multiple Roles of A Remarkable Hormone*. Sebastopol, California: BLL Publishing, 1993, 33.

10  Gittleman, A. L. *Super Nutrition for Menopause*. New York, New York: Simon and Schuster, 1993, 7-8.

11  Lee, L.. Ph. D. *Earthletter Newsletter* (June 1991)1:2.

12  Biskind, G.R. & Biskind, M.S. "Effect of B complex deficiency on inactivation of estrone in the liver." *Endocrinology* (1942) 31:109.

13  Cassidenti, D.L. et al. "Short-term effects of smoking on the pharmacokinetic profiles of micronized estradiol in post-menopausal women." *American Journal of Obstetrics & Gynecology* (1990): 163(6). Pt 1: 1953-1960.

14  Biskind, G.R. & Biskind, M.S. "Inactivation of testosterone propionate in the liver during vitamin B complex deficiency. Alteration of the estrogen-androgen equilibrium." *Endocrinology* (1945): 32:97.

15  Wyeth-Averst Laboratories. *Ladies Home Journal.* (February 1995):106.

16  Lee, J.R., M.D. *Natural Progesterone. The Multiple Roles of A Remarkable Hormone*. Sebastopol, California: BLL Publishing, 1993, 37.

17  Lauersen, N., M.D. & Whitney, S. *PMS Syndrome and You. It's Your Body*. Berkeley, California: Berkeley Books, 1983.

18  Hargrove, J.T., M.D. & Maxson, W.S., M.D. "Bioavailablility of oral micronized progesterone." *American Journal of Obstetrics & Gynocology* (1989): 161:4, 948-951. "Fertility and Sterility." 44:5,622-626. "Absorption of oral progesterone is influenced by vehicle and particle size. Menopausal hormone replacement therapy with continuous daily oral micronized estradiol and progesterone." *American Journal of Obstetrics & Gynocology* (1989): 73: 606-8.

19 Lee, J.R., M.D. *Natural Progesterone. The Multiple Roles of A Remarkable Hormone.* Sebastopol, California BLL Publishing, 1993, 52.

20 Lipshutz, A. *Steroid Hormones and Tumors.* Baltimore, Maryland: Williams and Wilkens Co., 1950.

21 Lemon, H.M., M.D. "Reduced estriol excretion in patients with breast cancer prior to endocrine therapy." *Journal of the American Medical Assocation* (1966): 196:120-36.

22 Cowan, L.D., et al. "Breast cancer incidence in women with a history of progesterone deficiency." *American Journal of Epidemiology* (1981):114:209.

23 Forman, J. "Navigating the maze of the estrogen replacement debate." *The Boston Globe.* (July 10, 1995): 25.

24 Whitehead, M.I et al. "The role and use of progestogens." *Obstetrics & Gynecology* (1990): 75(4)Suppl: 59S-76S Discussion 81S-83S.

25 Vandenbroucke, J.P. "Postmenopausal estrogen and cardio-protection." *The Lancet* (1991): 337:833-4.

## Chapter Four Notes

1 *The Soy Connection* (Fall 1994) 3:1.

2 Aldercreutz, H. et al. "Dietary phyto-estrogens and the menopause in Japan": *The Lancet,* (1992): 339:1233.

3 Peter-Welte C. et al. "Diesen" *Gynakol* (Germany), 1994: 7:1, 49-52.

4 Milewicz, A. et al. *Arzniem-forsch drug res.* (Germany), 1993: 43:7, 752-756.

5 Willard, T. *The Wild Rose Scientific Herbal.* Calgary, Alberta, Canada: Wild Rose College of Natural Healing, 1991, 343.

6 Duke, J. A., Ph.D. *Handbook of Medicinal Herbs.* 1985, 168.

7 Bergner. "Wild yam and hormonal synthesis." *Medical Herbalism* (Winter 1993): 4.

8 Chen, Y. & Wu, Y. "Progess in research and manufacturing of

steroidal sapogenins in China." *Journal of Herbs, Spices and Medicinal Plants* (1994): 2(3):59-70.

9  Willard, T. *The Wild Rose Scientific Herbal.* Calgary, Canada: Wild Rose College of Natural Healing, 1991, 343.

10  Lewis, W. & Memory, F. *Medical Botany.* Plants Affecting Mens Health, 318-319.

11  Lee, J.R., M.D. *Natural Progesterone. The Multiple Roles of A Remarkable Hormone.* Sebastopol, California: BLL Publishing, 1993: 4.

12  Northrup, C. *Women's Bodies, Women's Wisdom.* New York, New York: Bantam, 1994, 143.

13  Peat, R., Ph.D. Telephone interview, Minneapolis, March 1995.

14  Prior, J.C., M.D. "Progesterone as a Bone-trophics Hormone." *Endocrine Reviews.* (May 1990) 11:2:386-397.

15  Budoff, W. *No More Hot Flashes.* New York, New York: Warner Books, 1984, 7.

16  Budoff, W. *No More Menstrual Cramps and Other Good News.* Markham,Ontario: Penguin Books,1981.

## Chapter Five Notes

1  Peat, R. *Nutrition for Women.* Eugene, Oregon: Kenogen Publishers,1981, 27.

2  Frank, R. T. "The hormonal causes of premenstrual tension." *Archives of Neurologic Psychiatry* (1931): 26:1052.

3  Norris, R. "Progesterone for Premenstrual Tension" *Journal of Reproductive Medicine* (August 1983): 28: 8:511.

4  Biskind, G.R. & Biskind, M.S. "Effect of B complex deficiency on inactivation of estrone in the liver." *Endocrinology* (1942): 31:109.

5  Backstrom, T. and Carstensen, H. "Estrogen and progesterone in plasma in relation to menstrual tension." *Journal of Steroid Biochemistry* (1974): 5:257.

6  Chakmakjian, Z.H. "A critical assessment of therapy for the premenstrual tension syndrome." *Endocrinology and Metabolism and the Weinberger Endocrine Lab.* Baylor University Medical Center (August 1983): 8:532.

7  Abraham, G.E. "Premenstrual tension syndrome." *Obstetrics and Gynecology Nursing* (1980): 3:170.

8  Pizzorno, J. & Murray, M. *A Textbook of Natural Medicine.* Seattle, Washington: Bastyr College Publications, 1985.

9  Dalton, K., M.D. *Once a Month.* Emeryville, California: Hunter House, 1990, 21-22.

10 Dalton, K., M.D. *Once a Month.* Emeryville, California: Hunter House, 1990, 7.

11 "Thyroid Hypofunction in Premenstrual Syndrome" *New England Journal of Medicine* (December 4, 1986) 315:23:1486.

12 Lee, J.R., M.D. *Natural Progesterone. The Multiple Roles of A Remarkable Hormone.* Sebastopol, California: BLL Publishing, 1993, 47.

13 Greene R., and Dalton K. "The Premenstrual Syndrome" *British Medicine Journal* (1983) 1:10-071.

14 Lark, S. *The Estrogen Decision.* Los Altos, California: Westchester Publishing Company, 1994, 34.

15 Goei, G. S. Et al. "Dietary Patterns of Patients with Premenstrual Tension". *Journal of Applied Nutrition.* (1982) 34:4.

16 Lee, J.R., M.D. *Natural Progesterone. The Multiple Roles of A Remarkable Hormone.* Sebastopol, California: BLL Publishing, 1993, 47.

# Chapter Six Notes

1  Evans, B. *Life Changes: A guide to the menopause its effect and treatment.* London and Pan Books, 1992, 92.

2  Lark, S. *PMS: Premenstural Syndrome Self Help Book.* Berkeley, California: Celestial Arts Publishing, 1984, 55.

3  Bewley, S. and Bewley, T.H. "Drug dependence with oestrogen replacement therapy." *The Lancet* (1992): 339: 290-1.

4  Lee, J.R., M.D. *Natural Progesterone. The Multiple Roles of A Remarkable Hormone.* Sebastopol, California: BLL Publishing, 1993, 36.

5  Nielsen, F.H. "Nutritional requirements for boron, silicon, vanadium, nickel, and arsenic: current knowledge and speculation." *FASEB* (1991): 5:2661-2667.

6  Nielsen, F.H. et al. "Effect of dietary boron on mineral, estrogen, and testosterone metabolism in postmenopausal women." *FASEB* (1987): 1:394-397.

7  Nielsen, F.H. "Facts and fallacies about boron." *Nutrition Today* (May/June 1992): 6-12.

8  Reitz, R. *Menopause: A Positive Approach.* New York, New York: Penguin Books, 1979.

9  Harris, R.B. et al. "Are women using 11 postmenopausal estrogens? A community survey." *AJPH* (1990): 80(10):1266-1268.

10  Cassidenti, D.L. et al. "Short-term effects of smoking on the pharmacokinetic profiles of micronized estradiol in postmenopausal women." *American Journal of Obstetrics & Gynecology* (1990): 163(6). Pt 1: 1953-1960.

11  London, S. Et al. "Alcohol and other dietary factors in reation to serum hormone concentrations in women at climacteric." *American Journal of Clinical Nutrition* (1991): 53: 166-171.

12  Budoff, W. *No More Hot Flashes.* New York, New York: Warner Books, 1984, 7.

13  Lark, S. *PMS: Premenstural Syndrome Self Help Book.* Berkeley, California: Celestial Arts Publishing, 1984, 70.

14  Lee, J.R., M.D. *Natural Progesterone. The Multiple Roles of A Remarkable Hormone.* Sebastopol, California: BLL Publishing, 1993, 36.

15  Aldercreutz, H. et al. "Dietary phyto-estrogens and the menopause in Japan": *The Lancet,* (1992): 339:1233.

16 "American Journal Of Obstetrics And Gynecology August 1992 Study" quoted in *Preventive Magazine* (March 1993) 45:18

17 Youngs, D.D. "Some misconceptions concerning the Menopause, Sexuality, Depression" (1990): 75: 881-3. And Gath, D. And Iles, S. "Depression and the menopause." *British Medical Journal* (1990): 300: 1287-8.

18 Sheehy, G. *The Silent Passage*, New York, New York: Simon and Schuster, 1991, 7.

# Chapter Seven Notes

1 Tolstoi and Levin. "Osteoporosis, The Treatment Controversy", *Nutrition Today*, (July 8, 1992): 6-12.

2 Drinkwater, B. *Research Quarterly for Exercise and Sport* (1994):65:3:197 and Tory Hudson Interview.

3 Pruitt, L. A., et al. "Weight-training effects on bone mineral density in early postmenopausal women". *Journal of Bone and Mineral Research.* (February 1992): 179-185.

4 Zernicke, R., Professor of Kinesiology, UCLA. Reported at the 12th International Congress on Biomechanics, UCLA. (1989).

5 Barzel, U.S. "Acidic Loading and Osteoporosis." *Letters of the Journal of the American Geriatric Society* (1992): 30(9):613.

6 Draper, H. Et al. "Effects of high protein intake from common foods on calcium metabolism in postmenopausal women." *Nutrition Research* (1991): 11:273-81.

7 Recker, R.R. et al. "Effect of estrogen and calcium carbonate on bone loss in postmenopausal women." *Annuals of Internal Medicine* (1939): 87:649-655.

8 Pizzorno, J. & Murray, M. *A Textbook of Natural Medicine.* Seattle, Washington: Bastyr College Publications, 1985: 3.

9 Prior, J., M.D. "Progesterone and the prevention of osteoporosis." *Canadian Journal of OB/Gyn Women's Health Center* (1993):1(4):179.

10  Gambrell, R.D. Jr. "Estrogen replacement therapy and osteo-porosis." *Hospital Practice.* (1991):26 Suppl1:300-5.

11  Prior, J.C., M.D. "Progesterone as a Bone-trophics Hormone." *Endocrine Reviews.* (May 1990) 11:2:386-397.

12  Gaby, A., M.D., *Preventing and Reversing Osteoporosis.* Rocklin, California: Prima Publishing, 1994, 275.

13  Prior, J., M.D. "Progesterone and the prevention of osteo-porosis." *Canadian Journal of OB/Gyn Women's Health Center* (1993):1(4):179.

14  Lee, J. R., M.D. "The role of progesterone in the manage-ment of osteoporosis." *International Clinical Nutrition Review* (July 1990).

15  Lee J. R. M.D. "Is natural progesterone the missing link in osteoporosis prevention and treatment?" *Medical Hypotheses.* (August 1991): 35:4:316-8.

16  Lindsay, R. "Criteria for successful estrogen therapy in osteo-porosis." *Osteoporosis International* (1993): 3:Suppl 2:S9-12, Discussion S12-3. And "The effect of sex steroid on the skele-ton in premenopausal women." *American Journal of Obstetrics and Gynocology* (1993): 166:6:2.

17  Phillipe, E. Et al. "The endometrium under the effects of hormone replacement therapy in menopause with percu-taneios estradiol and low-dose micronized progesterone." *Pathologica* (Sep-Oct 1993): 85 (1099):475-87.

18  Hargrove, W. S., M.D. et al. "Absorption of oral progesterone is influenced by vehicle and particle size." *American Journal of Obstetrics and Gynocology* (October 1989): 161:4: 948-951.

19  Northrup, C. *Women's Bodies, Women's Wisdom.* New York, New York: Bantam, 1994, 454.

20  Mickelsen, O., and Marsh, A.G., "Calcium Requirement and Diet," *Nutrition Today* (Jan/Feb 1989): 28-32.

21  Barrest-Conner, E."Coffee-associated osteoprosis offset by daily milk consumption." *Journal of the American Medical Association* (1994) 26:2721:N4, 280(4)A.

22  Fuchs, J. Ph. D. "Factors in the Calcium Controversy."
    *Townsend Letter for Doctors* (Aug/Sept 1993): 906.

## *Herbal Materia Medica Notes*

1  Weiss, R.F. *Herbal Medicine.* England: Beaconsfield, 1988: 271.

2  Murray, M.T. *The Healing Power of Herbs.* Rocklin, California:
   Prima Publishing, 1995.

# Ordering Information

*I am interested in learning more about Melinda Bonk's discoveries.*

❏ Other titles from MB Publishers.

❏ How to order wild yam cream.

❏ Speaking to my organization _____ on _____

❏ Please call me right away! The best time to contact me is _____

❏ Please place my name on your mailing list for future information.

*You can order additional copies of this book by using this form.*

❏ Please send _____ copies of *Controlling Hormones Naturally,* at $12.95 each plus shipping and handling @ $2.00 per edition. (Minnesota residents only, add ___ Sales Tax of ___ per book) to:

NAME _____

STREET ADDRESS _____

CITY _____ STATE _____

ZIP CODE _____

TELEPHONE:

DAY _____ EVENING _____

My personal check or money order is enclosed, made payable to MB Publishers. All orders will be sent within 72 hours of receipt of good funds.

Quantity discounts for this book are available. Please call or write us today!

**MB Publishers**
**2101 Kennedy Street, NE, Suite 307**
**Minneapolis, MN 55413**
**Phone: (612) 378-8830**